Atlas of
PRACTICAL NEONATAL AND PEDIATRIC PROCEDURES

System requirement:

- Operating System—Windows XP or above.
- Web Browser—Internet Explorer 8 or above, Google Chrome, Mozilla Firefox and Safari.
- Essential plugins—Java and Flash player:
  - Facing problems in viewing content—it may be your system does not have Java enabled.
  - If Videos do not show up—it may be the system requires Flash player or need to manage Flash setting.
  - You can test Java and Flash by using the links from the troubleshoot section of the CD/DVD.
  - Learn more about Flash setting from the link in the troubleshoot section.

Accompanying CD/DVD ROMs are playable only in computer and not in DVD player.

CD/DVD has autorun function—it may take few seconds to load on your computer. If it does not work for you, then follow the steps below to access the contents manually:

- Click on my computer.
- Select the **CD/DVD drive** and click open/explore—this will show list of files in the **CD/DVD**.
- Find and double click file—"launch.html".

DVD Contents

Atlas of
PRACTICAL NEONATAL AND PEDIATRIC PROCEDURES

Pradeep Jain MD
Senior Consultant
Department of Anesthesiology
Pain and Perioperative Medicine
Sir Ganga Ram Hospital
New Delhi, India

Deepanjali Pant MD
Senior Consultant
Department of Anesthesiology
Pain and Perioperative Medicine
Sir Ganga Ram Hospital
New Delhi, India

Jayashree Sood MD FFARCS PGDHHM
Chairperson
Department of Anesthesiology
Pain and Perioperative Medicine
Sir Ganga Ram Hospital
New Delhi, India

Foreword
DS Rana

JAYPEE BROTHERS MEDICAL PUBLISHERS (P) LTD.
New Delhi • Panama City • London • Dhaka • Kathmandu

Jaypee Brothers Medical Publishers (P) Ltd.

Headquarters

Jaypee Brothers Medical Publishers (P) Ltd.
4838/24, Ansari Road, Daryaganj
New Delhi 110 002, India
Phone: +91-11-43574357
Fax: +91-11-43574314
Email: jaypee@jaypeebrothers.com

Overseas Offices

J.P. Medical Ltd.,
83, Victoria Street, London
SW1H 0HW (UK)
Phone: +44-2031708910
Fax: +02-03-0086180
Email: info@jpmedpub.com

Jaypee-Highlights Medical Publishers Inc.
City of Knowledge, Bld. 237, Clayton
Panama City, Panama
Phone: 507-301-0496
Fax: +507-301-0499
Email: cservice@jphmedical.com

Jaypee Brothers Medical Publishers (P) Ltd
17/1-B Babar Road, Block-B, Shaymali
Mohammadpur, Dhaka-1207
Bangladesh
Mobile: +08801912003485
Email: jaypeedhaka@gmail.com

Jaypee Brothers Medical Publishers (P) Ltd
Shorakhute, Kathmandu
Nepal
Phone: +00977-9841528578
Email: jaypee.nepal@gmail.com

Website: www.jaypeebrothers.com
Website: www.jaypeedigital.com

Inquiries for bulk sales may be solicited at: jaypee@jaypeebrothers.com

Atlas of Practical Neonatal and Pediatric Procedures

First Edition: **2013**

ISBN 978-93-5025-772-2

Printed at Ajanta Offset & Packagings Ltd., New Delhi.

Dedicated to

Our families, who believe that
we can and will overcome any adversity
through sheer hard work, strength
of character and love.
Their faith, courage and convictions are and
will always be an inspiration to us.

Foreword

Atlas of Practical Neonatal and Pediatric Procedures speaks for itself. Both anesthesiologists and pediatricians need to be updated regarding the airway management and resuscitation protocols in the pediatric population. This atlas has taken care of each such detail. The diagrams clearly depict with accuracy.

Each chapter of the book explains meticulously the different steps required to achieve optimal results. Most recent resuscitation guidelines have been included which are very essential for every practising anesthesiologist and pediatrician, whether he is an intensivist or not.

The Department of Anesthesiology, Pain and Perioperative Medicine, Sir Ganga Ram Hospital, New Delhi, India, is a centre of excellence, always at the forefront in clinical and academic activities.

DS Rana
Chairman
Board of Management
Sir Ganga Ram Hospital
New Delhi, India

Preface

There has been a long-felt need for the compilation of procedures done in the day-to-day practice of pediatric medicine, especially for the anesthesiologists, pediatricians, general practitioners and postgraduate students. This collection which is in the form of an atlas, broadly entails the common procedures applicable in pediatric patients and has been categorized into four divisions:

i. Airway management
ii. Vascular access
iii. Pain management
iv. Cardiopulmonary resuscitation (CPR) in neonates and children.

Airway management: In recent years, there has been an array of devices, techniques and improvizations for the improved and safe airway management in pediatric patients. We have covered most of the latest equipment and related guidelines.

Vascular access: Advancement of science has led to a better understanding of pediatric cardiovascular physiology and the recognition of the need for accurate and efficient hemodynamic monitoring. Therefore, the expertise in vascular access remains the cornerstone for intensive monitoring of the sick neonates and children. Various recent techniques and devices utilized for vascular access have been illustrated in a simplified way for easier perception and greater comprehensibility.

Pain management: The importance of pain management in neonates and infants for positive outcome, cost effectiveness, reduced hospital stay has now been substantiated. In this atlas, the emphasis is on the different regional techniques used for perioperative pain management and procedural sedation and analgesia in pediatric age group.

CPR in neonates and infants: The physiologic domain of CPR is rapidly expanding and so are the guidelines. The latest guidelines, at the time of printing the atlas, have been included.

The list of procedures detailed in this atlas is not all inclusive. We have tried to limit the atlas to the essentials.

Pradeep Jain
Deepanjali Pant
Jayashree Sood

Acknowledgments

At the very outset, we bow our heads to the Almighty who has blessed us abundantly, providing us with the necessary strength, courage and good health to bring this project to fruition.

We are grateful to Dr DS Rana, Chairman, Board of Management, Sir Ganga Ram Hospital, New Delhi, India, for his constant support and guidance.

We express our sincere gratitude to Dr Anil Jain, Dr Bimla Sharma, Dr Raminder Sehgal and Dr Chand Sahai for their contribution in providing the scientific material in preparing this atlas.

We are deeply indebted to our teachers Dr RS Saxena, Dr A Bhattacharya and Dr VP Kumra.

Our special thanks to our colleagues and postgraduate students, whose refreshing ideas, support and help made this mammoth of a task possible.

Our particular thanks to Mrs Silvi Philip and Mr Prakash Bisht for their secretarial help.

We are grateful to the colleagues in the Department of Pediatric Medicine and Pediatric Surgery for providing us with clinical material.

A heartfelt thanks to the academics department, especially to Mr Sansar and Mr Negi for their assistance in editing and preparing the videos.

We are also thankful to our families for their invaluable support and inspiration.

Contents

1 Airway Management

This chapter is designed to cover management of the pediatric airway under four subheadings:

A. Differences between pediatric and adult airway
B. Armamentarium of pediatric airway devices and associated equipment
C. Special airway techniques in children
D. Management of the difficult airway.

Normal Pediatric Airway

The area of greatest anatomic difference between an infant and an adult is in the airway **(Fig. 1.1)**.

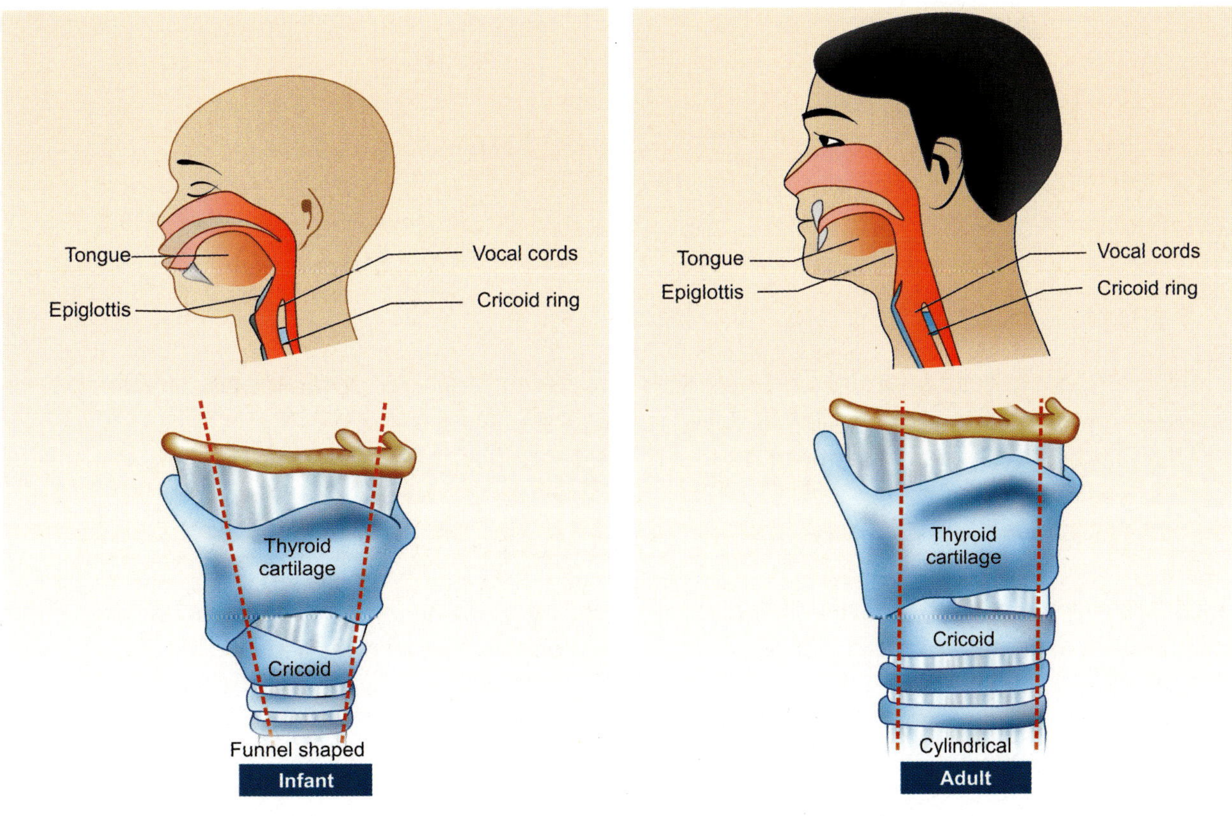

Fig. 1.1: Anatomical differences

Table 1.1: Anatomical differences and their significance

Parts	*Infant*	*Adult*	*Considerations in infant*
Head and neck	Large head, short neck, occipital protuberance	Normal	Hyperflexion of neck in supine position- a roll under the neck offsets this **(Figs 1.2A and B)**
Nares	Obligatory nasal breather, narrow nares, inclined floor of nasal cavity	Normal	Nasal secretions obstruct breathing Tongue contacts posterior wall of pharynx—obstructs airway
Tongue	Relatively large and posteriorly placed	Normal	Less roomy oral cavity – airway obstruction during mask holding Laryngoscopy and intubation more difficult
	Enlarged adenoids		Compounds airway obstruction
Epiglottis	Large, floppy, angled posteriorly over laryngeal inlet	Firm, less posterior angle	Control with laryngoscope blade more difficult. Folding of epiglottis during LMA insertion is frequent
Glottis	Anterior and higher, C_3 level in premature babies, C_3-C_4 level in newborn	C_5 level	Excess neck extension interferes with good visualization of glottis
Vocal cords	Inclined, slant anteriorly, prominent arytenoids	Flat	Insertion of endotracheal tube (ETT) more difficult especially for blind endotracheal intubation
Narrowest portion	Cricoid level	Glottis level	Significant while selecting size of ETT
Trachea	Short, mobile, posterior displacement into thorax	Long, stationary, vertical descent into thorax	Short trachea predisposes to accidental dislodgement of ETT or endobronchial intubation
Carinal angle	55 degrees both sides	25 degrees right and 45 degrees left side	Endobronchial intubation possible on either side
Lungs	Less elastic, smaller diameter of alveoli	Normal	Even a small amount of secretion can increase resistance
Diaphragm	Type II muscle fibers	Type I muscle fibers	Ability to perform repeated exercise is less, so respiratory muscle fatigue is common

Knowledge of these anatomical differences is essential for every practitioner to understand pediatric airway management **(Table 1.1)**.

The salient physiological differences are mentioned in **Table 1.2**.

Pediatric Airway Devices and Associated Equipment

There are many airway devices available to manage the pediatric airway. However, choosing the right airway device is a critical decision which depends on the experience and familiarity with the device.

These devices can be grouped into three main categories:

1. Face masks and airways
2. Tracheal tube and its alternatives
3. Conventional rigid laryngoscope and its alternatives.

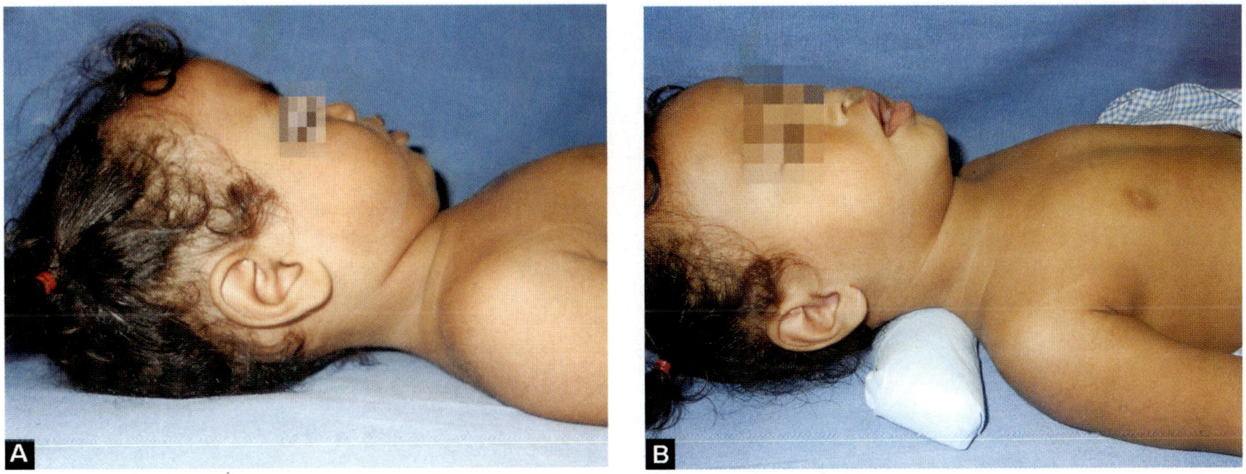

Figs 1.2A and B: Roll under neck: (A) Obstructed airway; (B) Patent airway

Table 1.2: Physiological considerations

Factors	*Infant*	*Adult*
O_2 Consumption	7 mL kg^{-1} min^{-1}	3.5 mL kg^{-1} min^{-1}
Minute ventilation	200 mL kg^{-1} min^{-1}	100 mL kg^{-1} min^{-1}
Respiratory rate	24–30 min^{-1}	10–15 min^{-1}
Pleural pressure	-1 to -2 cm H_2O	-5 cm H_2O
Vital capacity	35 ml kg^{-1}	70 ml kg^{-1}
FRC	30 ml kg^{-1}	35 ml kg^{-1}
Tidal volume	7 ml kg^{-1}	7 ml kg^{-1}
Dead space	2–2.5 ml kg^{-1}	2.2 ml kg^{-1}
Resistance to gas flow $\left(R \propto \frac{1}{r^4}\right)$	10 × of adults	Normal
pH	7.34–7.40	7.36–7.44
PaO_2 (mm of Hg)	60–85	85–95
$PaCO_2$ (mm of Hg)	30–36	36–44

FACE MASKS

The face mask is an essential adjunct for airway management in almost all situations. It is frequently used prior to laryngeal mask airway (LMA) or endotracheal tube (ETT) insertion and also for non-invasive positive pressure ventilation for treatment of respiratory failure. These masks are made up of non-conductive black rubber (neoprene), clear plastic or elastomeric material. Scented disposable PVC cushion face masks are commonly used in contemporary pediatric practice **(Fig. 1.3)**, but the anatomical black rubber face mask (Connell mask) is preferred in larger patients. Circular pediatric masks are available in silicone or black rubber versions **(Fig. 1.4)**.

The face mask has a body, a seal and a connector. A transparent body is more acceptable to the patient and also allows observation of vomitus, secretions, blood, lip color and exhaled

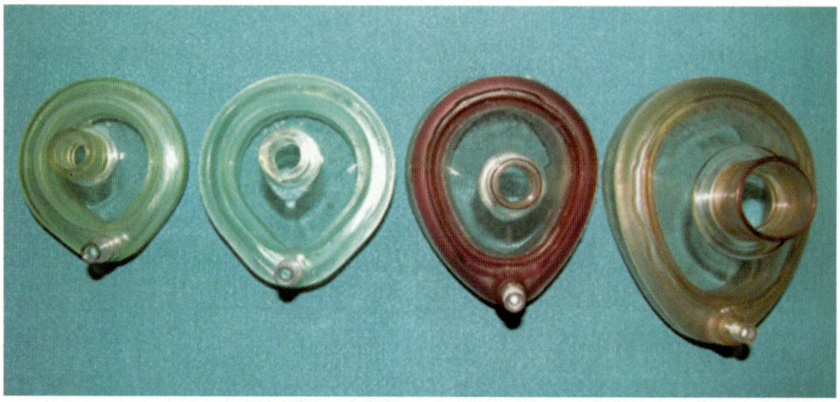

Fig. 1.3: Scented disposable PVC face masks

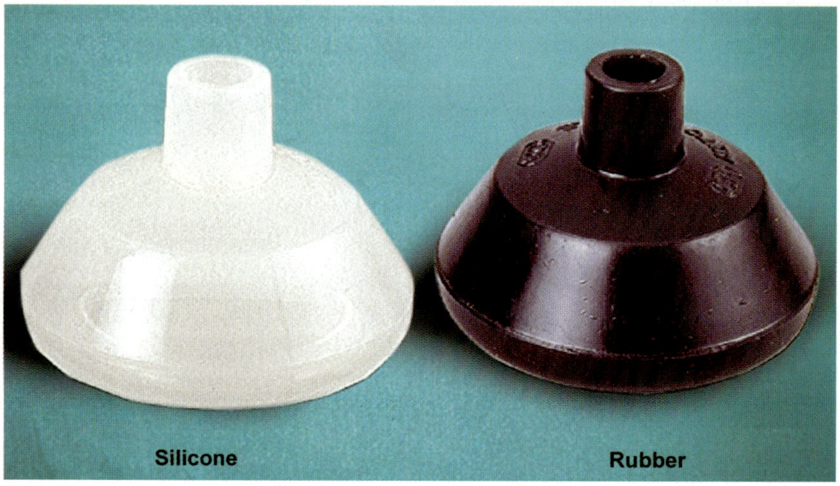

Fig. 1.4: Circular pediatric mask

moisture. The seal is either an air-filled cushion or a flap which conforms to the contour of the face. The connector part consists of a thickened fitting of ID 22 mm. A ring with hooks around the connector allows fixation with a harness or strap. The Rendell-Baker-Soucek (RBS) mask is specially designed for neonates and has a triangular body with minimal dead space (one quarter of the anatomical face mask) **(Fig. 1.5)**. It can also be used to achieve controlled or assisted ventilation over a tracheostomy stoma with its nasal end pointing caudally.

The endoscopic mask has a port for insertion of a fiberscope through nose or mouth while allowing simultaneous mask ventilation. The available sizes are usually for children more than four years of age **(Fig. 1.6)**.

Selection of a face mask of appropriate size and shape ensures a proper mask-fit for optimal ventilation with the least increase in dead space **(Table 1.3)**. The commonly used methods of holding a mask to maintain a patent airway with a tight seal are **(Figs 1.7A to C)**:

(i) One-hand method, (ii) Two-hand method, (iii) Claw-hand method.

i. *One-hand method (E-C clamp technique):* The thumb and index finger of the left hand are placed on the mask body to form a 'C' to hold the mask on the patients' face while the remaining three fingers are placed on the inferior surface of the mandible to form an 'E' to lift the jaw into the mask. Care should be taken to avoid pressure on the eyes and

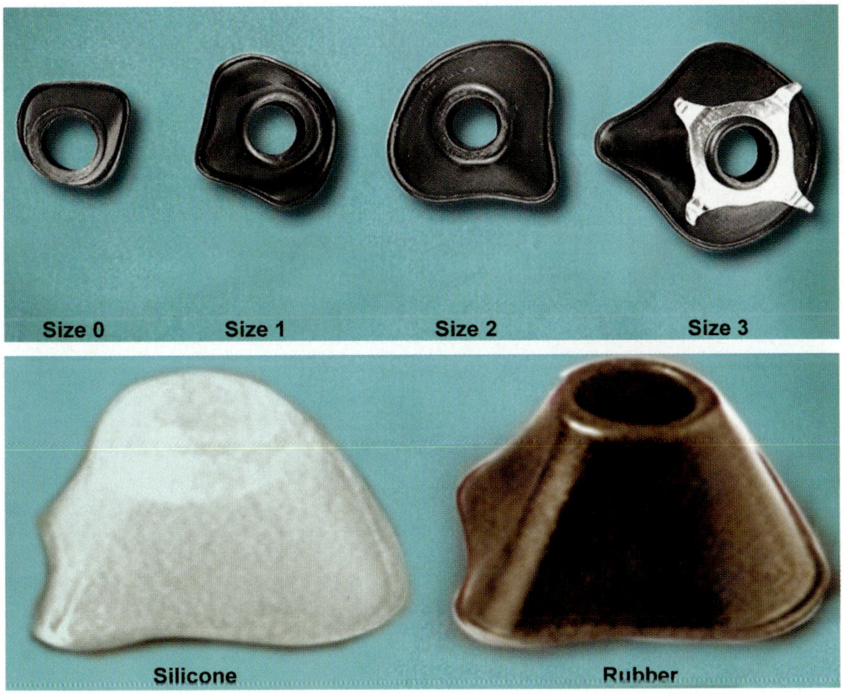

Fig. 1.5: Rendell-Baker-Soucek (RBS) masks

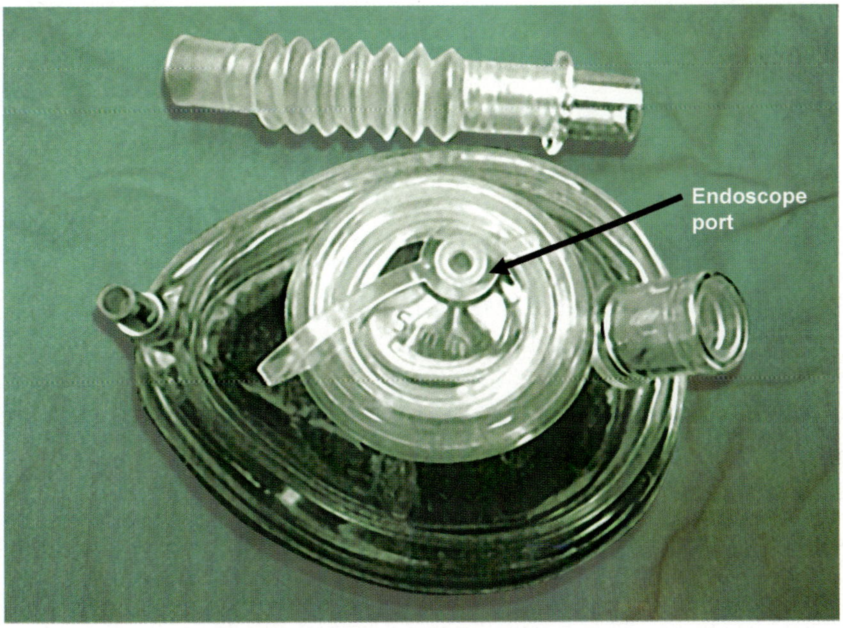

Fig. 1.6: Disposable endoscopic mask

compression of the submental soft tissues, since in young children the tongue can be pushed up to cause airway obstruction.

ii. *Two-hand method:* This method is used when the one-hand method is ineffective. A second person is required if manual assisted or controlled respiration is needed.
iii. *Claw-hand method:* This method is useful in short duration ophthalmic procedures where the anesthesiologist stands on the side facing the child. The face mask is applied in such

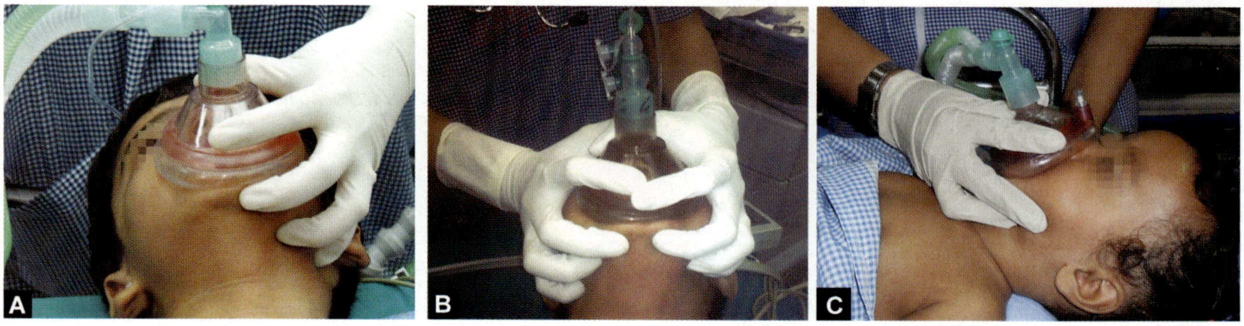

Figs 1.7A to C: Mask holding methods: (A) One-hand method; (B) Two-hand method; (C) Claw-hand method

a manner that the ring finger and middle finger go under the angle of the jaw on the opposite side and the thumb and index finger encircle the body of the mask to achieve a good seal. The palmar surface of the anesthesiologist's hand faces upwards unlike in the previous methods where it faces downwards.

Table 1.3: Different types of face masks

Age group	*Rendell-Baker-Soucek mask*	*Circular mask*
Premature	0	00
Infant	1	0
Small child	2	0A
Child	3 with hook	0B

Advantages

- Lower incidence of sore-throat
- Requires less anesthetic depth
- Cost-efficient method to manage the airway for short cases.

Disadvantages

- User fatigue
- Higher fresh gas flow required
- Not useful in remote anesthesia (i.e. MRI/CT scan)
- More episodes of oxygen desaturation
- $PaCO_2$-$EtCO_2$ gradient higher particularly with small tidal volume because of large dead space ventilation
- May require more frequent intraoperative airway manipulations
- Work of breathing increases during spontaneous breathing.

Complications

- Gastric inflation during controlled ventilation
- Skin allergy to the material or residue from chemical or gas sterilization
- Eye injury due to ill-fitting mask and undue pressure applied
- Nerve injury due to pressure from mask or strap, stretching from extreme forward jaw displacement or unstable cervical spine.

AIRWAYS

Airways lift the tongue and epiglottis away from the posterior pharyngeal wall thus preventing obstruction of the space above the larynx. Airways always require a face mask as a ventilatory device and decrease work of breathing during spontaneous respiration. The airway may be inserted via the oral or nasal route. The nasopharyngeal airway is used in a pediatric patient with gag reflex while an oropharyngeal airway is for patients without gag reflex. Sizing of the airway is in the same way as for an adult. Measurement landmarks are from the corner of the mouth or nose to the tip of the ear lobule.

Complications

- Airway obstruction by the tongue or epiglottis due to incorrect size or improper insertion
- Trauma to nose, lip, tongue, teeth and pharynx
- Tissue edema, ulceration and necrosis of nose or tongue when airway is *in situ* for an extended period
- Coughing and laryngospasm if airway is introduced during inadequate depth of anesthesia.

Oropharyngeal Airways

These are made of PVC or elastomeric material. Each airway has a flange at the buccal end to prevent over-insertion. The bite portion is straight, fits between the teeth or gums and is reinforced to prevent occlusion by biting. The curved portion extends backwards to correspond to the shape of the tongue and palate. Oral airway insertion does not cause movement of cervical spine. The oral airway does not need to be inverted when inserted into the mouth of an infant or small child. It should never be inserted in case of epiglottitis as total airway obstruction may be precipitated. The most popular oral airway is the Guedel airway which has its bite-portion color-coded according to size **(Fig. 1.8)** **(Table 1.4)**. The dual channel design of Berman oral airway allows access of a suction catheter and a color coded version is also available for easy identification **(Fig. 1.10)**.

Table 1.4: Sizes available for pediatric age group (Fig. 1.9)

Age group	*Color code*	*Order size*	*Length (mm)*	*ISO size*
Newborn	Transparent	000	30	3
	Pink	00	40	4
Children	Blue	0	50	5
	Black	1	60	6
	White	2	70	7

Advantages

- Maintains an open airway
- Facilitates oropharyngeal suctioning

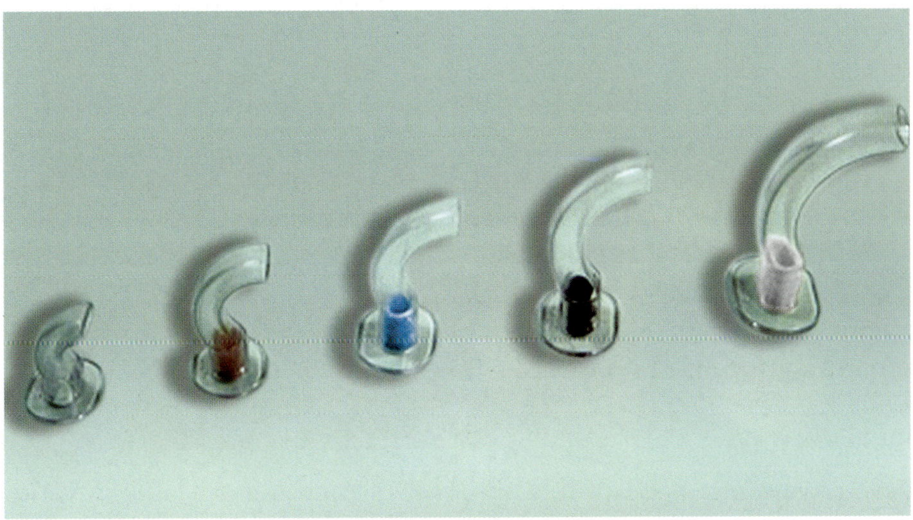

Fig. 1.8: Guedel oropharyngeal airways

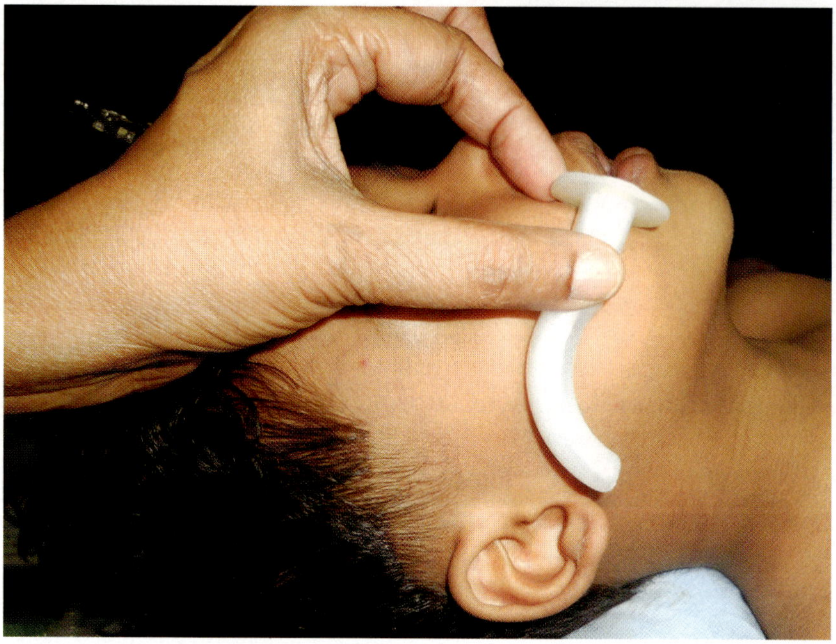

Fig. 1.9: Sizing of oral airway

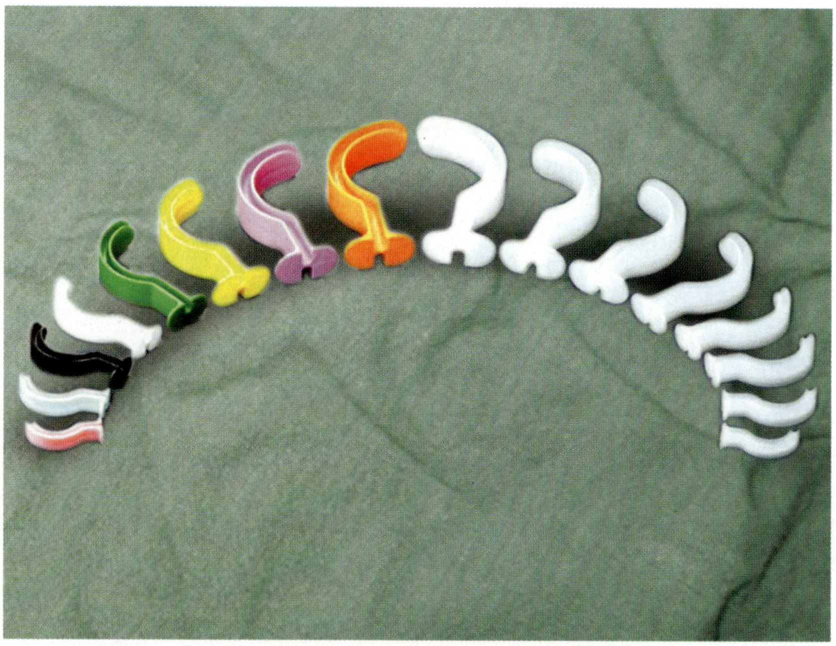

Fig. 1.10: Berman oropharyngeal airways

- Protects tongue or orotracheal tube from being bitten
- Provides a pathway for inserting device into pharynx or esophagus.

Nasopharyngeal Airways

Nasopharyngeal airways are made of rubber or plastic and are available in various sizes **(Figs 1.11A and B)**. The anatomic constraints of the nasal passages limit the scope for various designs of nasal airways. Most consist of a flange and a curved cylindrical tube. The flange,

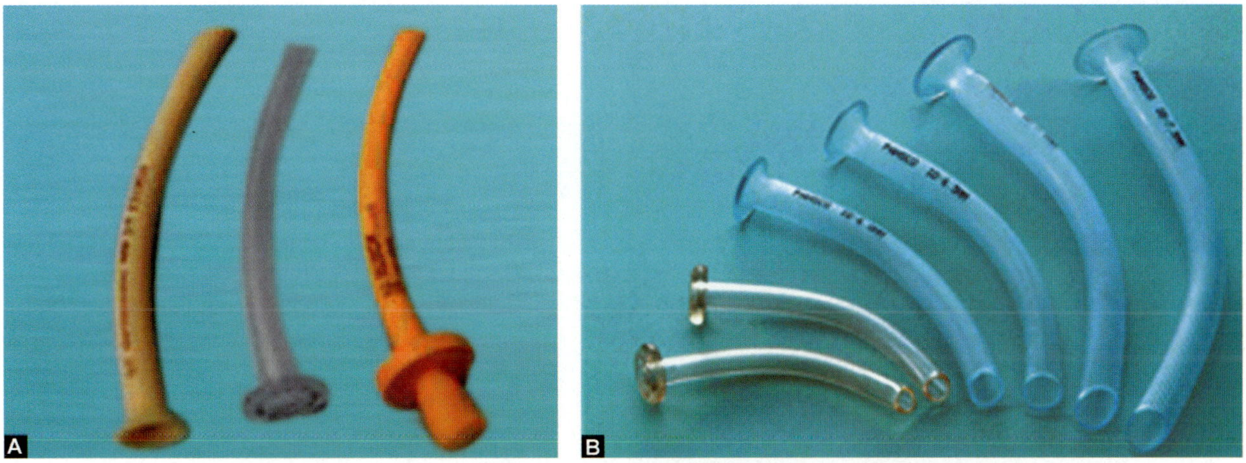

Figs 1.11A and B: (A) Nasopharyngeal airways; (B) Different sizes of disposable nasal airways

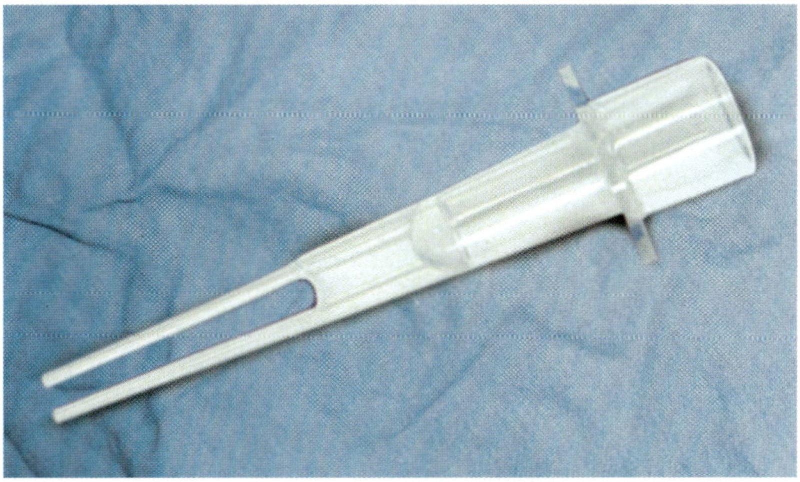

Fig. 1.12: Binasal airway

sometimes aided with a safety-pin, prevents it from slipping deep into the nose. The tube is curved to follow the anatomic shape of the nasal floor and nasopharynx. Most nasal airways are uncuffed and use one nostril, but some are cuffed. A binasal airway consists of two nasal airways joined together by an adapter for attachment to a breathing system or CPAP machine **(Fig. 1.12)**.

Nasal airway should be lubricated thoroughly along its entire length. A vasoconstrictor may be applied to the nostril before insertion of airway to reduce trauma. Insert the airway gently without resistance, in a perpendicular direction with the curve oriented towards the mouth. Too deep an insertion may stimulate the laryngeal reflex and too short an insertion may not relieve airway obstruction. Ideally, when fully inserted, the pharyngeal end should be below the base of the tongue, but above the epiglottis **(Table 1.5)**. The ideal size is 0.5-1 mm smaller than the appropriate orotracheal tube. Nasopharyngeal airway is available in sizes 2 to 8.5 mm which indicate the internal diameter in millimeters **(Fig. 1.13)**.

Indications

- Situations where access to the mouth is limited
- Avoidance of the oral cavity is desirable (loose /bad dentition, lingual frenulum)

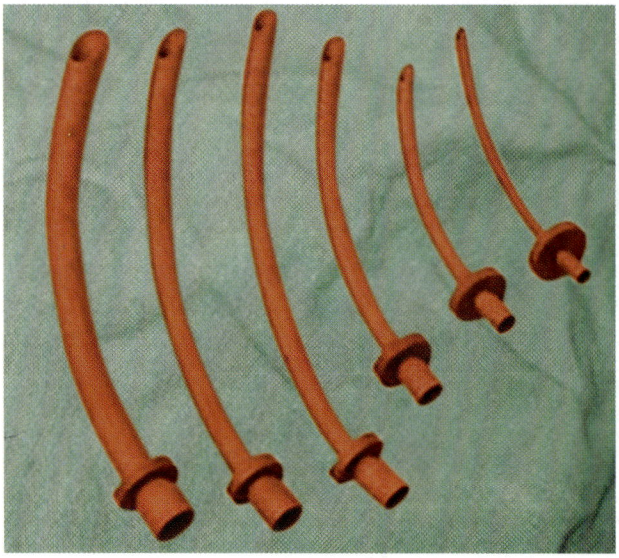

Fig. 1.13: Different sizes of nasal airways with adjustable flange

Table 1.5: Size of nasal airways with adjustable flange (Fig. 1.14)

Size/ID (mm)	*OD (mm)*	*Length (mm)*
2	4	
2.5	4.7	95
3	5.3	
3.5	6	
4.5	6.7	125
5	7.3	
5.5	8	170
6	8.7	

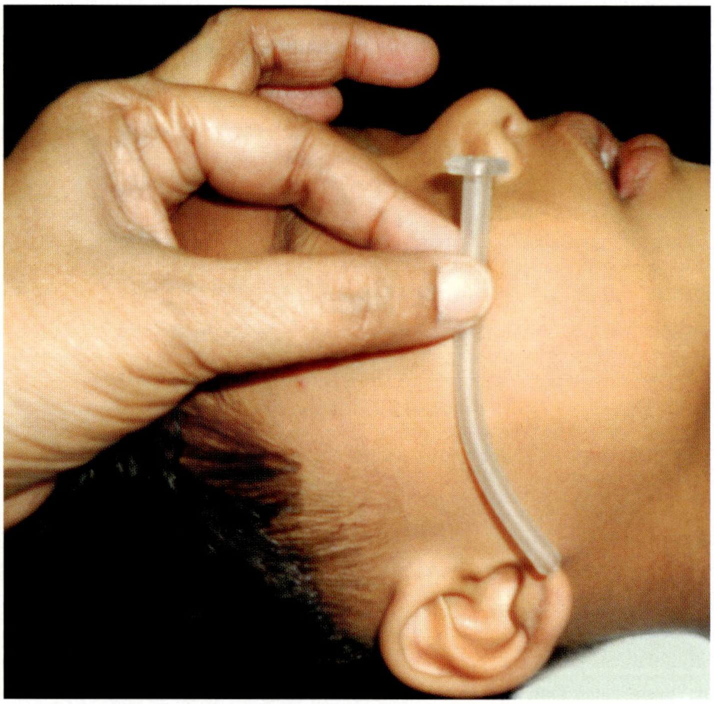

Fig. 1.14: Sizing of nasopharyngeal airway

- Useful back-up when orally inserted airway fails
- Awake, semi-comatose or lightly anesthetized patients—better tolerated and less easy to dislodge
- Cuffed nasal airway for ventilation
- Guidance of fiberoptic instruments, suction catheters, and nasogastric tube into the laryngopharynx.

Contraindications
- Nasal pathology
- Fracture base of the skull
- Bleeding disorders
- Large adenoids or tonsils.

AIRWAY DEVICES

Airway devices can be further divided into:
a. Supraglottic devices
b. Infraglottic devices.

SUPRAGLOTTIC DEVICES

These cuffed devices are inserted blindly via the oral route, to secure airway in case of elective or emergency situations. The tip of the device sits in the hypopharynx and its cuff or base forms a seal incorporating the supraglottic area. These devices can be used for spontaneous as well as positive pressure ventilation, but do not provide adequate protection against aspiration. They can be further grouped as:
1. Laryngeal mask airway (LMA)
2. Non-LMA supraglottic devices
   a. Cuffed oropharyngeal airway
   b. Laryngeal tube and laryngeal tube suction device
   c. Cobra perilaryngeal airway
   d. Combitube.

Laryngeal Mask Airway

The LMA is the most frequently used and tested supraglottic airway device. It consists of a curved shaft and an elliptical spoon shaped cup surrounded by an inflatable cuff with an inflation tube along with a self-sealing pilot balloon **(Fig. 1.15)** **(Table 1.6)**.

The LMA family now includes a variety of LMAs and the advanced use of special purpose LMAs requires an impeccable technique and good communication with the operating

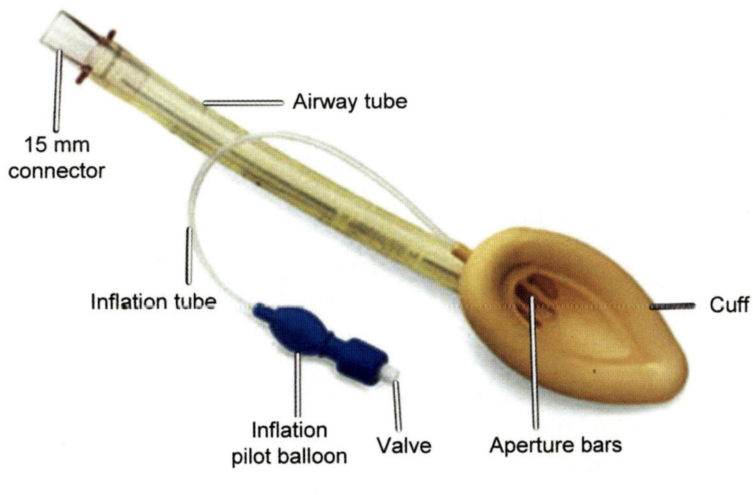

Fig. 1.15: Parts of laryngeal mask airway (LMA)

Table 1.6: Cuff volume and size of LMA

Mask size	*Patient size*	*Maximum cuff volume (ml)*	*Largest ETT (ID) mm*	*Largest fiberscope (ED) mm*
1	Neonates (<5 kg)	4	3.5	2.7
1.5	Infants (5–10 kg)	7	4.0	3.0
2	Child (10–20 kg)	10	4.5	3.5
2.5	Child (20–30 kg)	14	5.0	4.0
3	Child (30–50 kg)	20	6.0 cuffed	4.5

surgeon **(Table 1.7)**. Too large a size is difficult to place whereas too small a size predisposes to gas leak during positive pressure ventilation.

One size smaller and one size larger than the chosen size should always be immediately available. The inflating syringe should be dry and contain only air. Method of insertion can be the *classic insertion* with deflated cuff or partially deflated with the *lateral insertion* technique or with mask opening facing the palate till base of tongue is bypassed and then rotated 180° into the final position. Since there is no statistical difference between the different methods of LMA insertion, it is better to change to another when one method is not working.

Advantages

- Easy insertion
- Reliable performance
- Less invasive than intubation
- Decreased incidence of trauma, sore throat
- Facilitates smooth emergence
- Cost-effective as requires lesser anesthetic depth.

Disadvantages

- Epiglottic downfolding
- Malpositioning
- Inadequate protection against aspiration.

Uses

- Provides airway under anesthesia during elective operative procedures, for spontaneous or controlled ventilation
- In procedures outside the operating room such as GI endoscopy, flexible bronchoscopy, interventional radiology, radiation therapy
- As a conduit for ETT in the management of the difficult airway
- Provides airway during resuscitation (ASA guidelines)
- Conduit for drug administration (i.e. surfactant to neonate with respiratory distress syndrome)
- Useful alternative for airway control in children with an upper respiratory infection.

Cuffed Oropharyngeal Airway (COPA)

This supraglottic device is a modified Guedel oral airway with a cuff at its distal end, which creates a seal between the patient's upper airway and the anesthesia delivery system **(Fig. 1.29)**. When the cuff is inflated, it displaces the base of the tongue anteriorly and passively elevates the epiglottis away from the posterior pharyngeal wall. The proximal end has a standard

Table 1.7: Supraglottic devices (LMA family)

S. No.	Name	Description	Size (Pediatric use)	Clinical application	Special features
1.	Classic LMA (1991) **(Figs 1.16A to E)**	Original prototype, made up of silicone, latex-free, reusable upto 40 times	5 sizes (1, 1.5, 2, 2.5, 3)	Maintenance of airway	Soft silicone cuff – Less chance of throat irritation and stimulation
2.	LMA Unique (1997) **(Fig. 1.17)**	Disposable classic LMA, made up of medical grade PVC	5 sizes (1, 1.5, 2, 2.5, 3)	Used where a reusable device not practical or economical (infective cases in OR, ambulance, ER, crash carts)	Stiffer tube and less compliant cuff-ideal to warm it prior to use to make it softer. Intracuff pressure increases less with use of N_2O in comparison to classic LMA
3.	LMA ProSeal (PLMA) (2000) **(Figs 1.18A to E)**	Most versatile member of LMA family – Airway tube shorter, narrower – Integral drain tube with opening at tip allows passage of a gastric tube and venting of gastric gas and liquid – Integrated bite–block – Bowl deeper, no bar – Cuff softer and larger proximally, higher sealing pressure – Second dorsal cuff present in sizes $\geq$ 3	5 sizes (1, 1.5, 2, 2.5, 3)	Preferred in controlled ventilation	Reusable, autoclavable – Facilitates PPV, provides airway protection Method of insertion: a. Introducer tool method b. Finger – insertion method c. Guided method (stylet/bougie/ fiberscope) in difficult airway
4.	LMA Supreme (2008) **(Fig. 1.19)**	Disposable PLMA Made up of PVC and polycarbonates, anatomically shaped airway tube—easy insertion	Size 3 for children 30-50 kg	Situations where reusable device not advisable	Hybrid of PLMA and ILMA Smaller sizes are currently under development
5.	Flexible LMA (1993) **(Fig. 1.20)**	Longer, narrower, flexible wire-reinforced shaft, but cuff size is same. – Available in both reusable and disposable version – More difficult to insert, may require a stylet to stiffen	3 sizes (2, 2.5, 3)	Adenotonsillectomy, oral surgery, head and neck surgery, ophthalmic and dental procedures, radiation therapy Unsuitable for MRI/prolonged spontaneous ventilation (due to narrow tube)	Less likely to be displaced during head rotation or tube repositioning – Kink-proof, but does not prevent obstruction from biting. – Malposition less easily diagnosed as tube does not give clear indication of cuff orientation

Contd...

Contd...

S. No.	*Name*	*Description*	*Size (Pediatric use)*	*Clinical application*	*Special features*
6.	Intubating LMA (ILMA, Fastrach) (1997) **(Fig. 1.21)**	Mask attached to a rigid stainless steel short tube curved to align the aperture to glottis – Attached metal handle aids one-handed insertion, adjustment and stabilization during ETT insertion – Does not need finger insertion into mouth	Size 3 for 30-50 kg (can accommodate 6 mm ETT)	True pediatric size requires the curve to be re-configured to fit airway in a small child – Unsuitable in MRI unit – Adequate mouth opening with difficult laryngoscopy (high anterior larynx) – For ventilation – To aid intubation (blind/ visually guided)	Single, movable epiglottic elevating bar present – Available in silicone/disposable version – ETT is non-disposable, silicone – reinforced, high pressure low volume cuff, not for prolonged use – Expensive
7.	LMA C-Trach (2005) **(Fig. 1.22)**	Similar to ILMA, but with two built-in fiberoptic channels which emerge under epiglottic bar. One channel transmits light, the other conveys image to monitor at proximal end attached via a magnetic latch connector	Same as ILMA	Awake intubation – Very useful in unstable cervical spine – Indication and insertion technique same as ILMA	Battery operated, rechargable – Autoclavable upto 20 times – Real-time image of glottis – improves first-attempt intubation rate
8.	Soft seal LMA **(Fig. 1.23)**	Similar to LMA unique but large oval cuff, deeper bowl, no tapering at tip. No epiglottic bar, clear shaft allows easier visualization of secretion and exhaled condensation Embedded blue pilot line exits proximally, so remains out of way and less irritation	Size and cuff volume same as classic LMA	Disposable, cost-effective, eliminates risk of cross-infection – Easy access for flexible fiberoptic devices	– made of PVC – less permeable to N_2O – pilot balloon labeled with size and maximum cuff volume
9.	Ambu LMA **(Fig. 1.24)**	Cuff tapered at the tube. Extra-soft cuff, reinforced tip does not bend during insertion, no aperture bar	Size and cuff volume same as classic LMA	Disposable, cost-effective in infected cases – Reusable version also available	Shaft larger, more rigid and precurved which replicates human anatomy, especially in smaller babies
10.	LMA classic Excel **(Fig. 1.25)**	Similar to classic LMA, soft silicone cuff, removable connector for easy fiber-optic assisted intubation	Size 3 for 30-50 kg	6.5 mm cuffed ETT can be negotiated	Maximum cuff inflation volume up to 20 ml

Contd..

Contd...

S. No.	*Name*	*Description*	*Size (Pediatric use)*	*Clinical application*	*Special features*
11.	Solus LMA **(Figs 1.26A to C)**	Includes standard, MRI compatible and flexible tube LMA	Size and cuff volume same as classic LMA	Disposable	MRI compatible – ferrous free option with MRI logo
12.	I-gel **(Figs 1.27A and B)**	Named after the unique soft –gel like material (SEBS: Styrene Ethylene Butadiene Styrene) of which it is made up – Epiglottis blocker present – Buccal cavity stabilizer aids insertion and prevents rotation – Gastric channel and integral bite block enhances safety	Four sizes (1, 1.5, 2, 2.5)	Both for spontaneous or controlled ventilation – In sniffing position, glide it downwards and backwards along hard palate with a continuous but gentle push until a definitive resistance is felt –	Easy to use and a safe and rapid airway management solution, less trauma – Single use, latex-free – No cuff inflation is required, so avoids compression trauma – No finger insertion is required – Color coded polypropylene 'protective cradle' Size 1 without gastric channel
13.	Intubating Laryngeal Airway (ILA) **(Fig. 1.28)**	A dark blue oval bowl with a clear curved silicon tube. Hypercurved airway tube approximates anatomy, Easy insertion Opening into bowl has ridges on top and sides to prevent trapping of epiglottis. Ridges below outlet improves mask seal	Disposable sizes (1, 1.5, 2, 2.5) Reusable size (2.5)	– Primary airway – Aid for intubation in difficult airway situation	– Autoclavable upto 40 times – Downward tilt at tip of bowl helps to slip below epiglottis – Keyhole shaped airway outlet directs the ETT in midline towards the laryngeal inlet, facilitates intubation – Reusable removal stylet available in 2 sizes which allows controlled removal of ILA after intubation

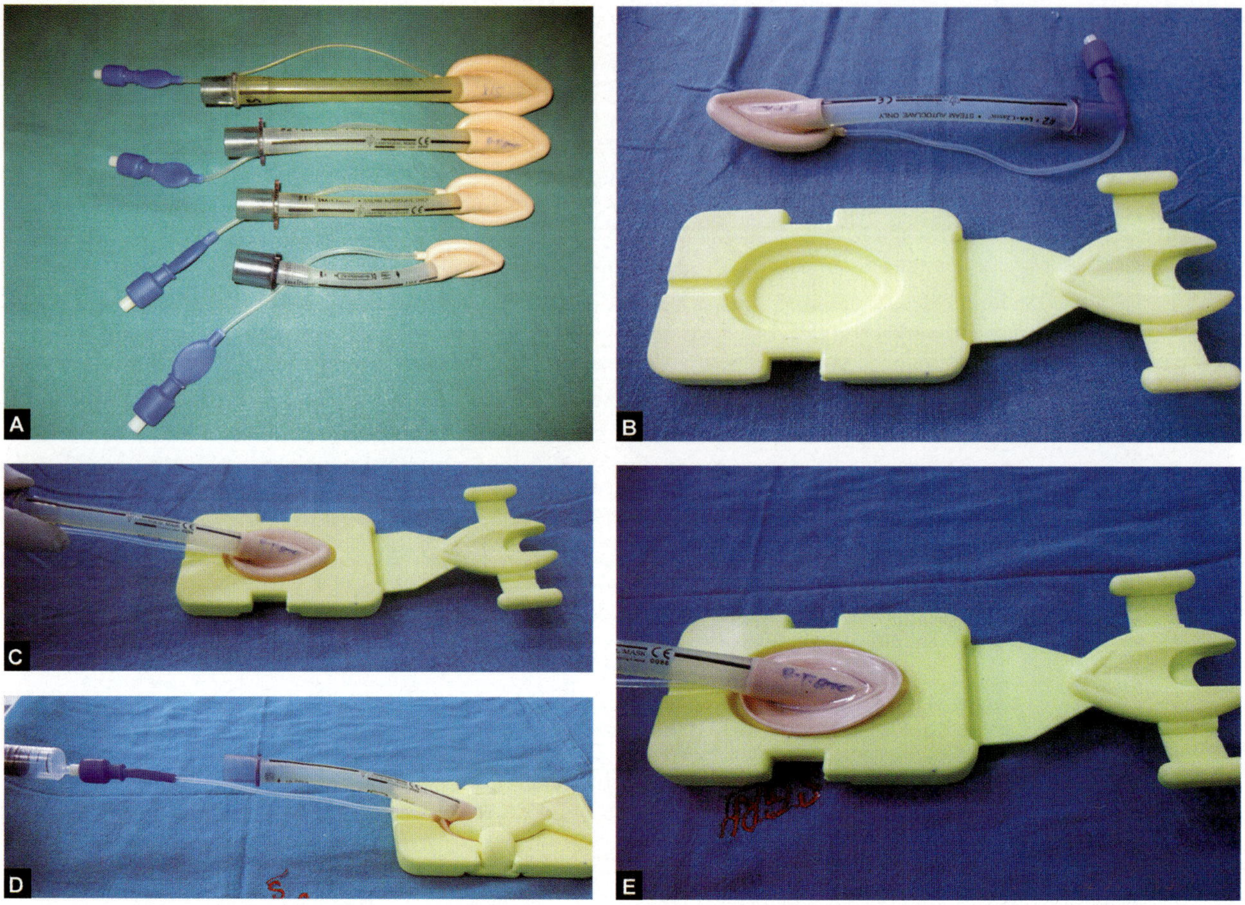

Figs 1.16A to E: (A) Classic LMA (sizes 1, 1.5, 2, 2.5); (B to E) Technique of using deflator

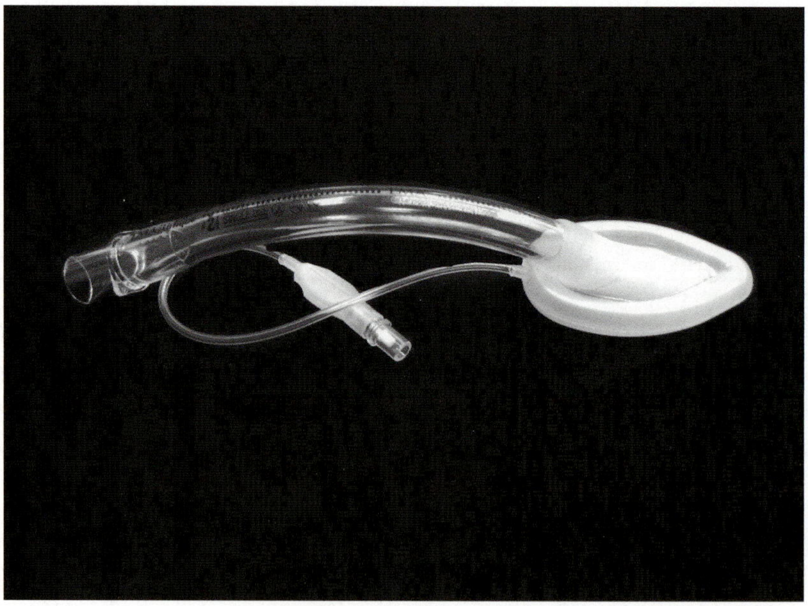

Fig. 1.17: LMA-unique

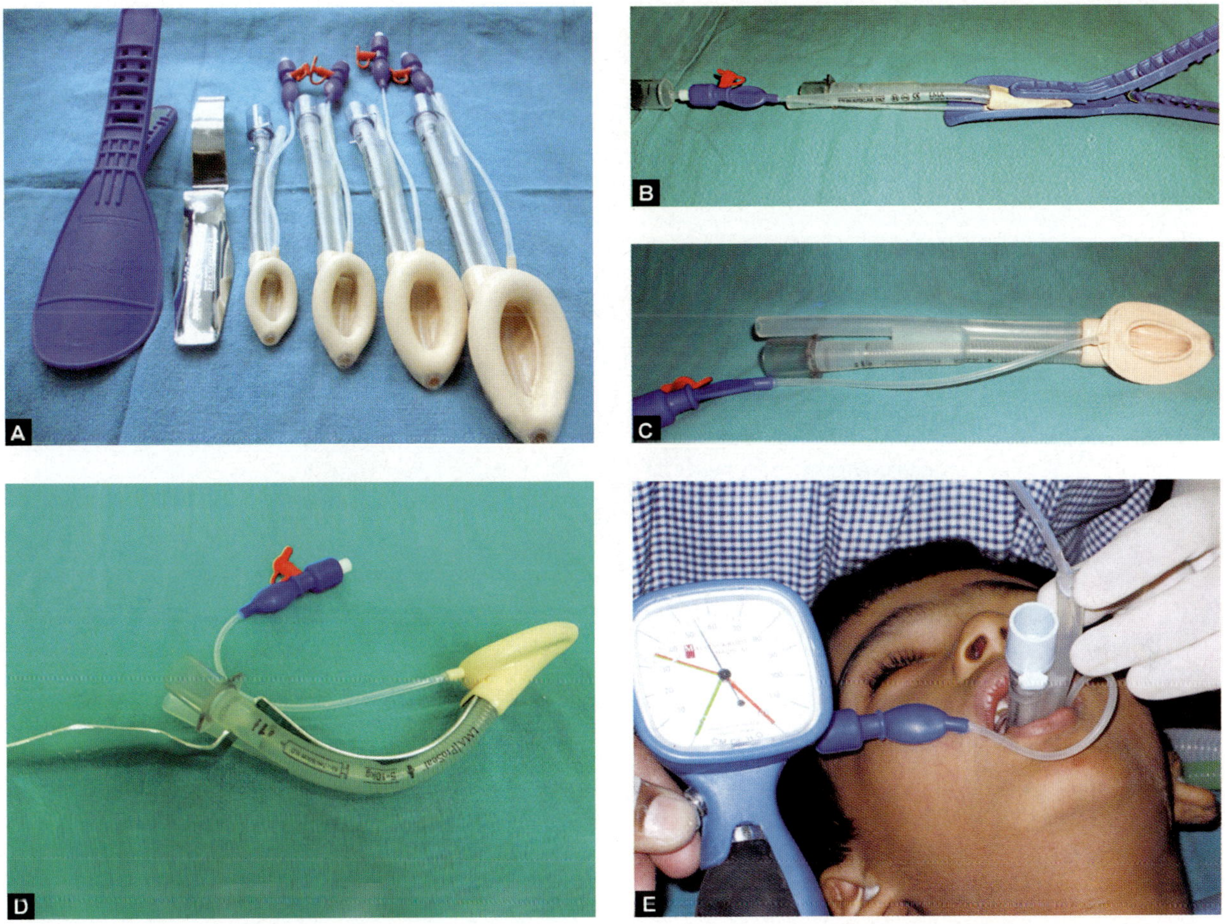

Figs 1.18A to E: (A) LMA ProSeal (sizes 1, 1.5, 2, 2.5); (B) PLMA with cuff deflator; (C) PLMA with deflated cuff; (D) PLMA with introducer; (E) PLMA *in situ* with cuff pressure measurement

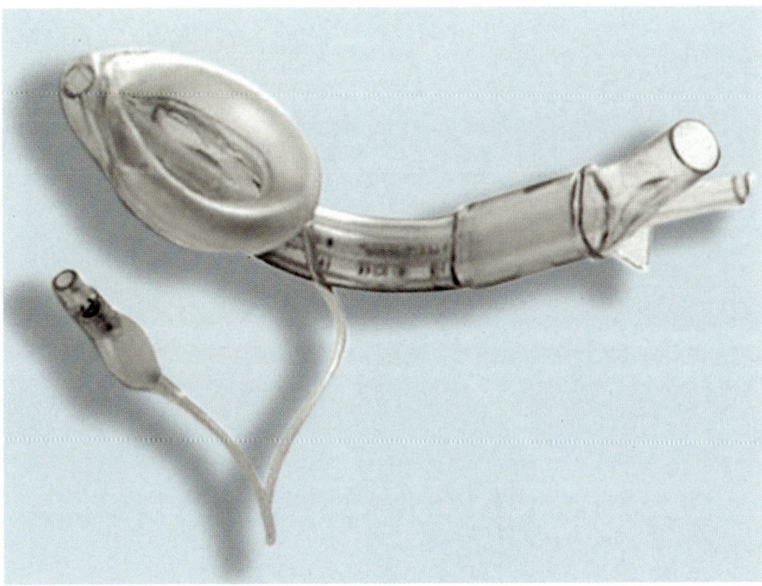

Fig. 1.19: LMA supreme

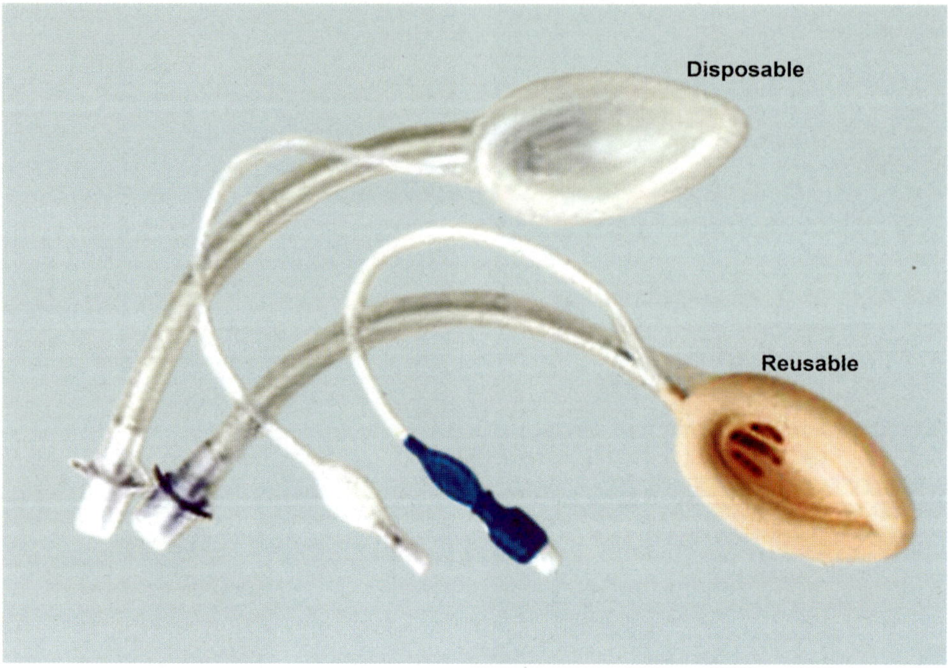

Fig. 1.20: Flexible LMA

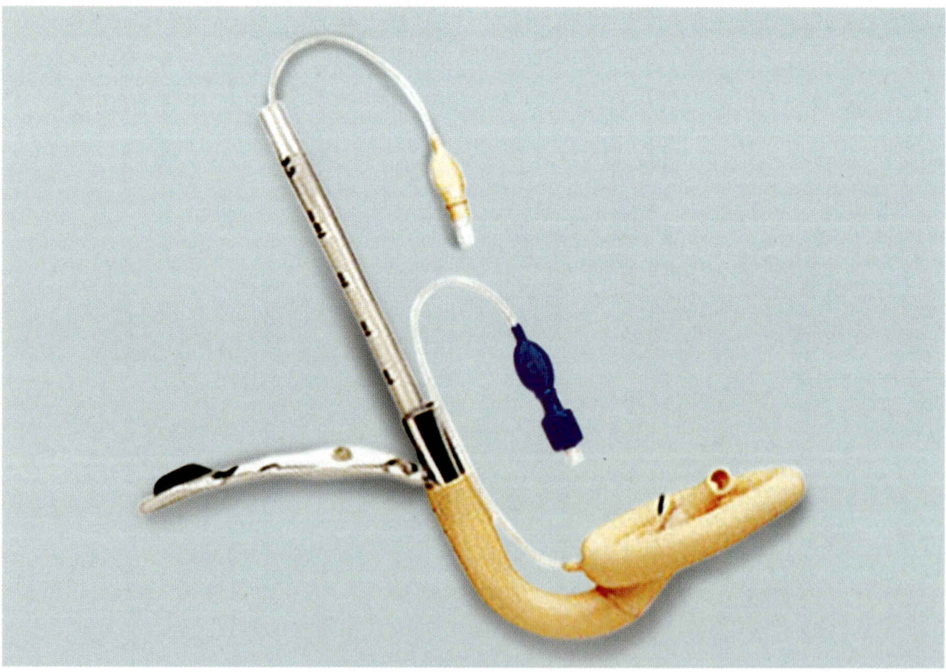

Fig. 1.21: Intubating LMA

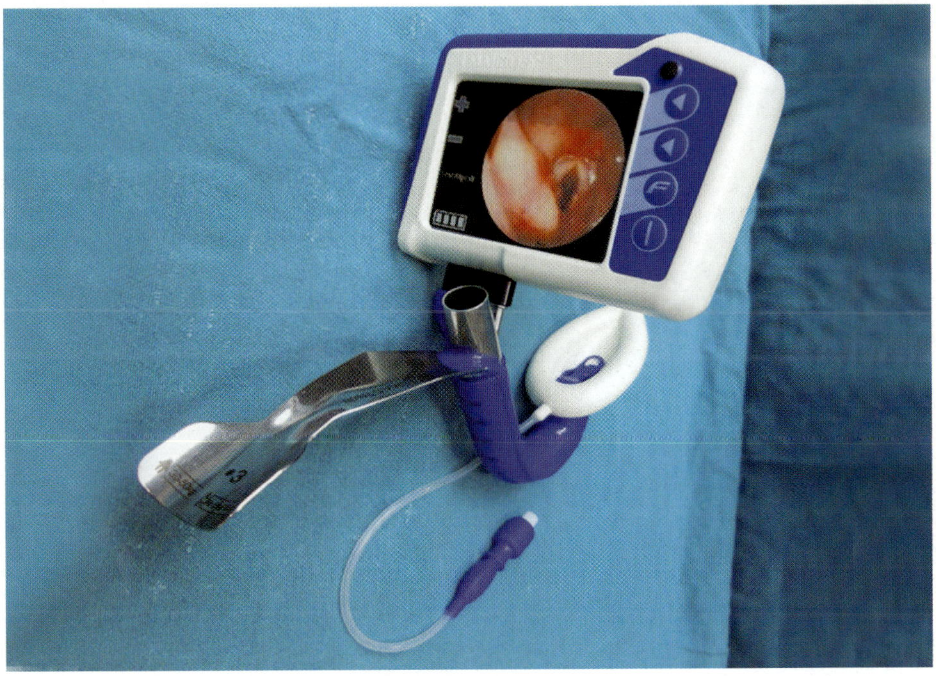

Fig. 1.22: LMA C-trach

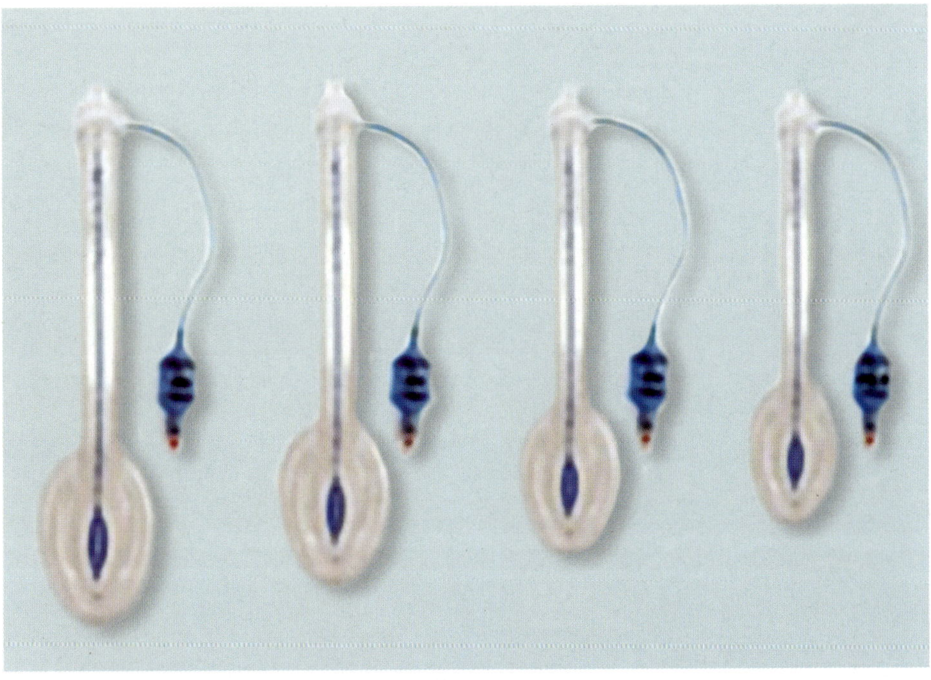

Fig. 1.23: Soft seal LMA (sizes 1, 1.5, 2, 2.5)

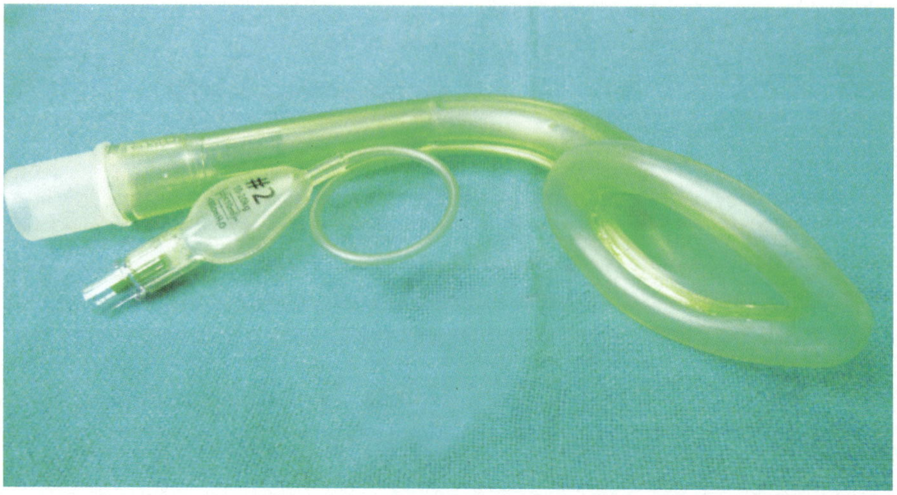

Fig. 1.24: Disposable ambu LMA

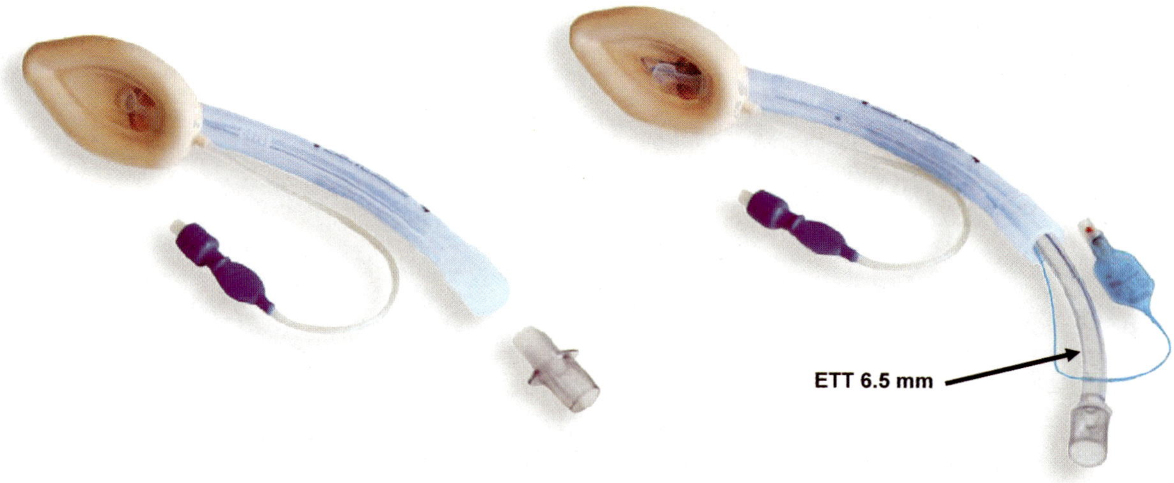

Fig. 1.25: LMA classic excel

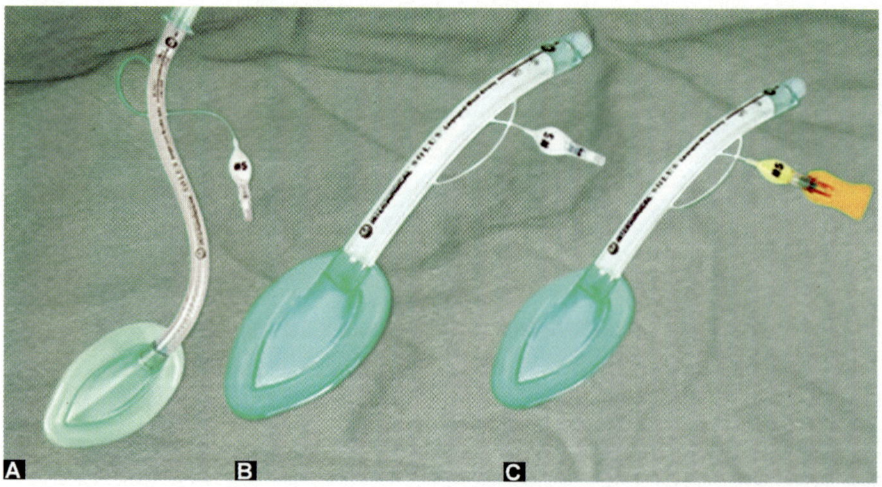

Figs 1.26A to C: Solus LMA: (A) Flexible; (B) Standard; (C) MRI compatible

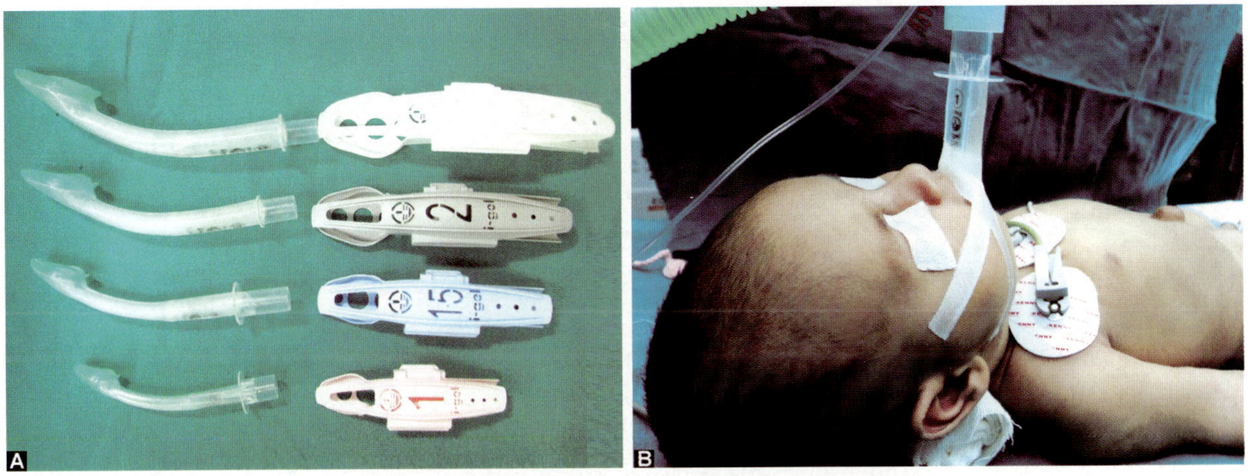

Figs 1.27A and B: (A) I-gel; (B) I-gel *in situ*

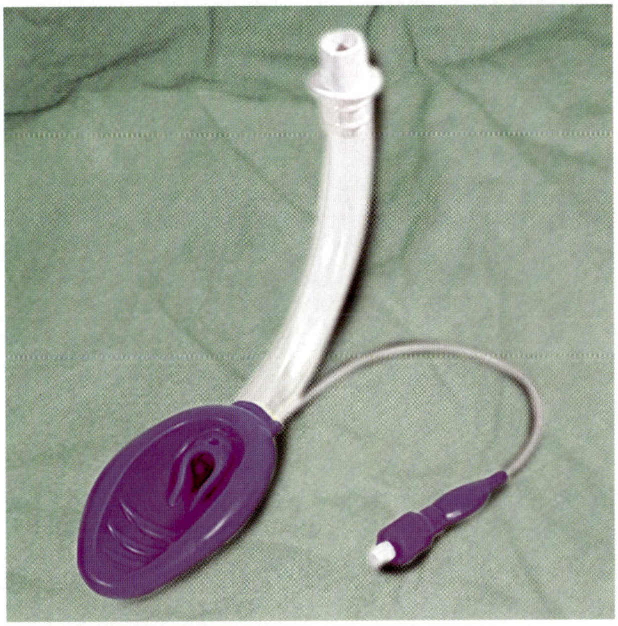

Fig. 1.28: Intubating laryngeal airway

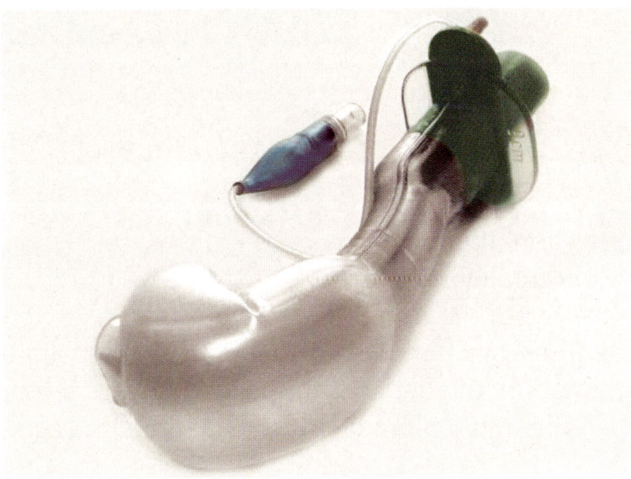

Fig. 1.29: Cuffed oropharyngeal airway (COPA)

15 mm connector for connecting the device to the anesthesia circuit, an integrated bite-block (tooth-lip guard) and two posts for attaching the elastic fixation strap. The number of sizes available refers to the distance in centimeters between the tooth-lip guard and the distal tip. The bite block is color coded for size. The smallest size available is suitable for bigger children only **(Table 1.8)**.

Table 1.8: Sizes of COPA

Size	*Color*	*Volume of air*
8	Green	25 cc
9	Yellow	30 cc
10	Red	35 cc
11	Light green	40 cc

Cuffed oropharyngeal airway (COPA) size can be determined by measuring the distal tip of the device at the angle of the jaw with the COPA perpendicular to the patient's head (as for oral airway). Selecting the right size is the most important step in using the COPA. The technique of insertion is the same as that for an oral airway. After insertion the COPA should be strapped with colored bite block between the teeth in the midline. Then the jaw thrust/chin lift is done and cuff is inflated with the appropriate volume of air.

Indication: Obese pediatric patients with small mouth undergoing general anesthesia with spontaneous ventilation for minor surgery or any painful procedure.

Advantages
- Easy insertion even in inexperienced hands
- Less anesthetic depth required when compared to LMA
- Allows hands free anesthesia.

Disadvantages
- Frequent airway manipulations may be necessary intraoperatively
- Not suitable for controlled ventilation as the airway seal pressure is low.

Laryngeal Tube (LT)

This newly developed supraglottic device consists of a relatively wide and curved single lumen tube with two anterior facing, oval-shaped ventilation outlets in between its two low pressure high volume cuffs—a large proximal oropharyngeal cuff near the middle of the tube and a small distal esophageal cuff near the blind distal tip.

It is available in both reusable (silicone) and disposable (PVC) versions. It is available in six sizes with color coded connector according to size. One inflation tube inflates both light blue cuffs simultaneously. The approximate inflation volume is indicated on syringe with color coding **(Table 1.9)**.

Table 1.9: Sizes of LT/LTS for pediatric age-group (Figs 1.30A and B)

Size	*Max. cuff volume (ml)*	*Color of connector*	*Patient size*
0	10	Transparent	Neonate < 5 kg
1	20	White	Infant 5-12 kg
2	35	Green	Child 12-25 kg
2.5	60	Orange	Child 125-150 cm

In neutral or sniffing position, the fully deflated device is inserted in midline and slid along the palate into the hypopharynx until resistance is felt. The three black marks on the shaft should align with the upper incisors (thicker middle line for orientation, thinner lines for eventual repositioning). The cuffs are inflated to a pressure of 60 cm H_2O. The inflated proximal cuff stabilizes the tube and blocks oropharynx and nasopharynx.

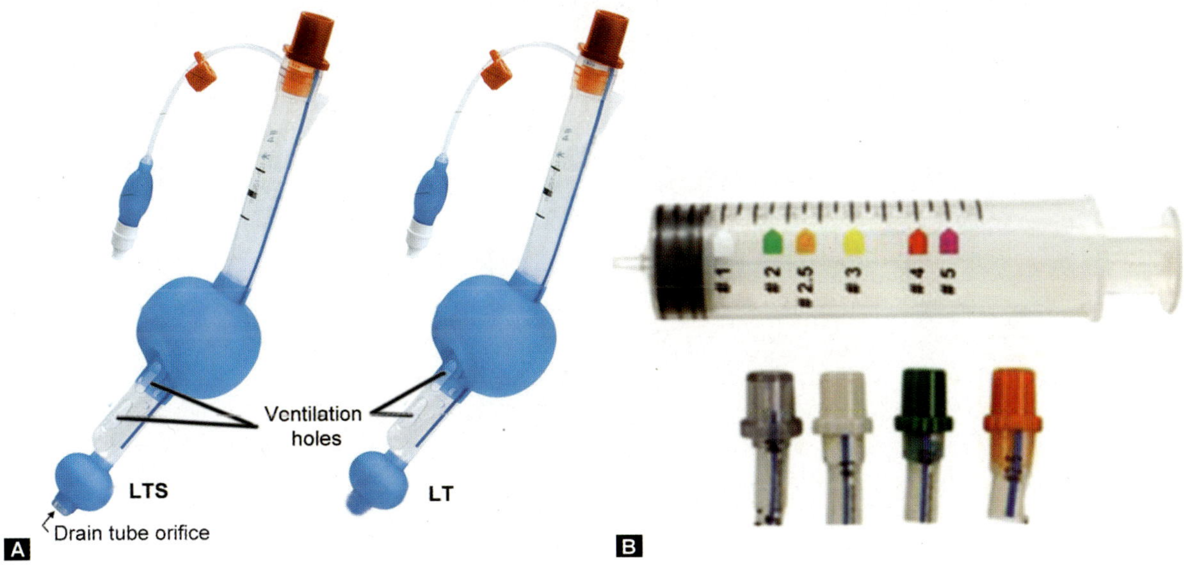

Figs 1.30A and B: (A) LT and LTS; (B) Color coded connector and syringe

Advantages
- Easy insertion
- Useful for both spontaneous and controlled ventilation
- Ventilatory holes act as a guide for airway exchange catheter placement or fiberscope and also allow suction.
- Risk of gastric inflation is low as distal cuff blocks esophageal inlet, so protects against aspiration
- Higher ventilation pressure can be used when required
- Especially useful for resuscitation in the difficult airway scenario
- Low laryngopharyngeal morbidity.

Disadvantages
- PLMA proves superior to LT
- In manual in-line neck stabilization, ILMA proves superior to LT.

Laryngeal Tube Suction (LTS) Device

This device is identical to LT in terms of its size and method of insertion. It is available in both reusable and disposable version. It has an additional (esophageal) lumen posterior to the respiratory lumen that ends just distal to the esophageal cuff for suction and gastric tube placement. LTS has been recommended as the first line device to secure the airway in a difficult airway. However, as with all supraglottic devices, familiarity and clinical experience with the device and its insertion technique is essential for safe and successful use, especially in an emergency.

Cobra Perilaryngeal Airway (Cobra PLA)

This disposable supraglottic device is a single lumen breathing tube with a wide, tapered distal end (cobra head design). It has a low pressure, high volume, oval cuff attached just proximal to

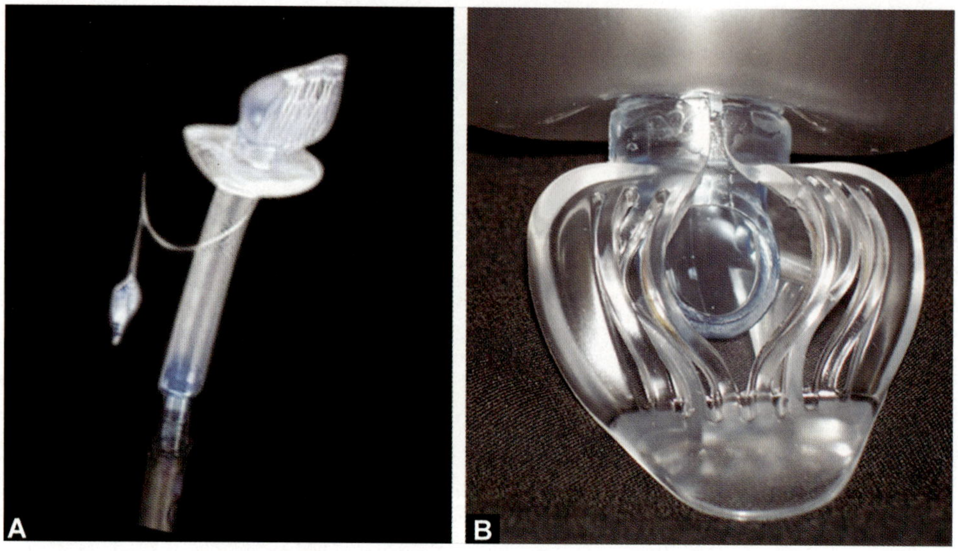

Figs 1.31A and B: (A) Cobra perilaryngeal airway; (B) Distal end

the wide part. It is termed perilaryngeal because when positioned in hypopharynx, the distal end abuts the aryepiglottic folds and directly sits on the laryngeal inlet. The distal ventilatory end has a unique design such that the series of slots prevent the ventilatory hole from being obstructed by the epiglottis and soft tissue **(Figs 1.31A and B)**.

Inflation of cuff to a pressure less than 25 cm H_2O seals off the distal end from the upper airway and allows positive pressure ventilation. The device is available in eight sizes, out of which five sizes are for pediatric age group **(Table 1.10)**.

Table 1.10: Pediatric sizes of Cobra PLA

Size	*Patient weight (kg)*	*Tube (ID/mm)*	*Cuff volume (ml)*	*ETT (ID/mm)*
0.5	>2.5	5.0	<8	3.0
1.0	>5	6.0	<10	4.5
1.5	>10	6.0	<25	4.5
2.0	>15	10.5	<40	6.5
3.0	>35	10.5	<50	6.5

With the patient in a sniffing position, the deflated and lubricated device is inserted in midline back into the mouth (not towards the hard palate) until resistance is felt. The cuff is inflated with enough air to obtain an adequate seal.

Advantages

- Useful alternative in "Cannot ventilate cannot intubate" (CVCI) situation
- Easy insertion, less sore throat
- Large lumen as a conduit for ETT or fiberscope
- Short breathing tube allows ETT to pass below vocal cords without removing it.

Disadvantages

- No protection against aspiration
- Cuff leak
- Possible airway obstruction.

Esophageal Tracheal Combitube (ETC)

It is a disposable double-lumen tube that combines the features of a conventional ETT and that of an esophageal obturator airway. It has a large proximal latex oropharyngeal balloon and a

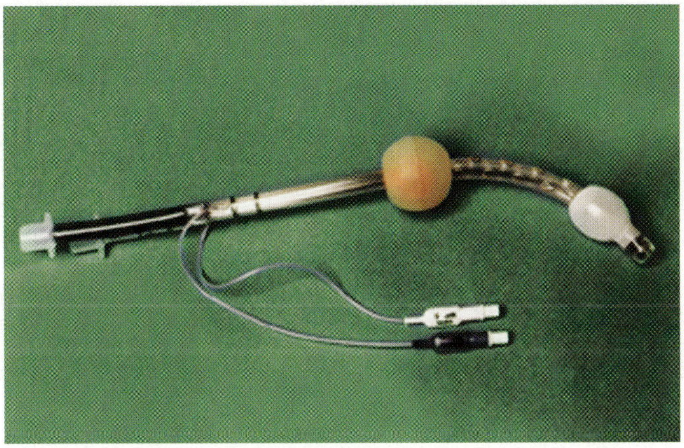

Fig. 1.32: Esophageal tracheal combitube (ETC)

distal esophageal low-pressure cuff with eight ventilatory holes in between. Ventilation is possible with either tracheal or esophageal intubation **(Fig. 1.32)**. It can be inserted blindly, quickly and with a relatively low level of skill. It enters the esophagus in 99% of insertions. It reduces the likelihood of aspiration.

Indications
- Elective or emergent situations, both in and out of hospital environment
- Situations where neck movement is contraindicated
- Limited access to airway
- CVCI situation
- Massive airway bleeding or regurgitation.

Limitation
- The smallest (37 F) size can only be used in children taller than 4 feet.

INFRAGLOTTIC DEVICES

These include: (a) Endotracheal tubes, (b) Tracheostomy tubes.

Endotracheal Tubes (ETTs)

Traditionally, uncuffed tracheal tubes were routinely used in children. They are available for both nasal and oral use in various sizes, the smallest being 2 mm ID. In recent years, cuffed tracheal tubes are preferred, mostly in small children, especially in the pediatric ICU and emergency department **(Fig. 1.33) (Table 1.11)**.

Cuffed Endotracheal Tube

Advantages
- Less gas leak around tracheal tube
- Reduced need to exchange inappropriately sized ETT
- More consistent ventilation
- Ventilation with higher inspiratory pressure possible
- Decreases risk of aspiration
- Less use of oversized uncuffed tube

Table 1.11: Size of ETT and Depth of insertion

Age	*Weight (kg)*	*Size (mm)*	*Depth (cm)*
Premature newborn	< 1	2–2.5	7
< 3 months	1-2	3	8
3-9 months	2-3	3.5	9
> 9 months		$\frac{\text{Age(years)} + 16}{4}$	

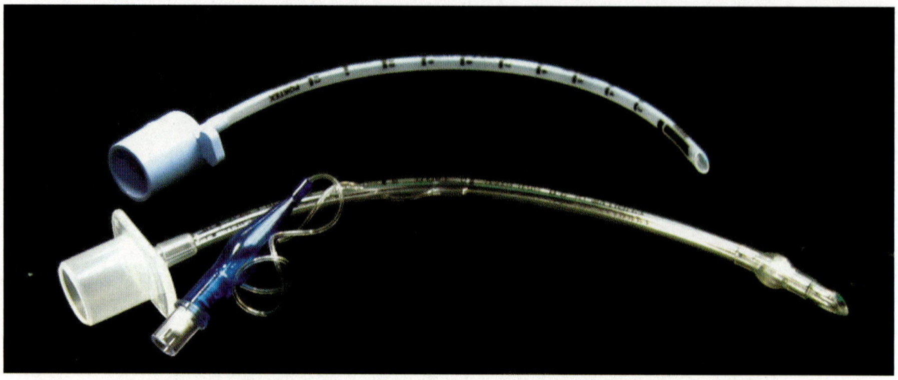

Fig. 1.33: Endotracheal tube ID 3 mm (cuffed and uncuffed)

- Low flow anesthesia
- More reliable end-tidal carbon dioxide monitoring
- Reduces atmospheric pollution.

Disadvantages

- Cuff hyperinflation leading to tracheal mucosal injury
- Risk of post extubation stridor
- Reduced ID of tube—higher resistance and work of breathing, difficulty in suctioning
- Frequent cuff pressure monitoring is required
- Subglottic stenosis.

Ultra thin high-volume, low-pressure polyurethane cuff results in lower sealing pressure than the conventional cuff. There are considerable differences in the outer tube diameter for a given ID and in length of cuff from different manufacturers. A pressure of 20 cm H_2O is sufficient to provide a seal without compromising tracheal mucosal blood flow, which is compromised at 30 cm H_2O and completely obstructed at 45 cm H_2O.

When the child's age is unknown, the tube size approximates to the external diameter of distal phalanx of little finger or diameter of external nares. Age is recognized as the most reliable indicator of appropriate ETT size selection.

Penlington's Formula:

$< 6\frac{1}{2}$ years → ETT (mm) = Age (yr)/3 + 3.5

$> 6\frac{1}{2}$ years → ETT (mm) = Age (yr)/4 + 4.5

ETT half a size larger and half a size smaller than calculated should be available as well. Cuffed ETT should always be half size smaller than the above calculated uncuffed diameter.

Depth of insertion (cm) oral:

a. $\frac{\text{Age (yr)}}{2} + 12$

b. $\frac{\text{Weight (kg)}}{5} + 12$

c. $\frac{\text{Height (cm)}}{10} + 5$

d. 3 × ETT (ID in mm)

Rule of 7-8-9-10 in infant (depth of insertion at lips):

I kg-7 cm, 2 kg-8 cm, 3 kg-9 cm, 4 kg-10 cm

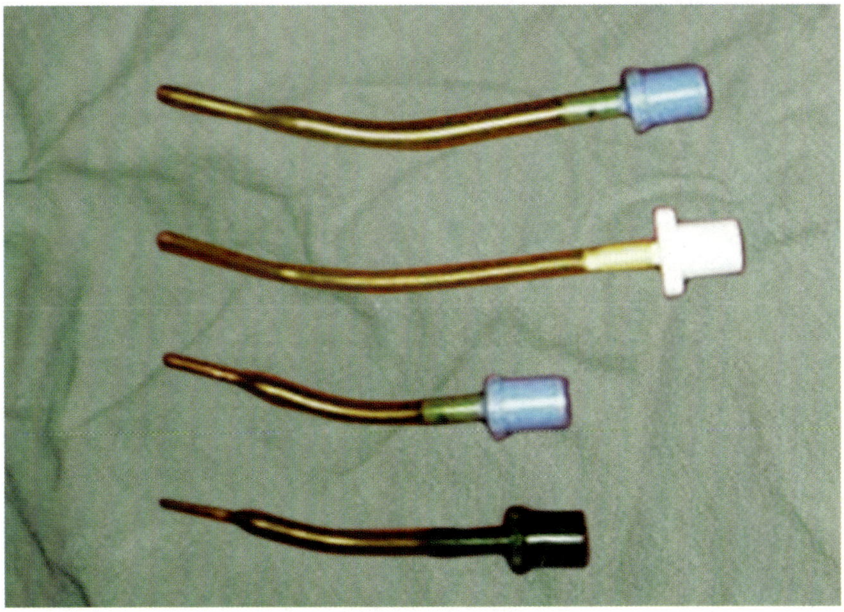

Fig. 1.34: Cole tube

The desired depth of a nasotracheal tube is 20% more than oral tube. The practical formula is simplified as nasal tube depth = oral depth + 2 cm.

SPECIAL TYPES OF ETT

Cole Tube (Fig. 1.34)

Its distal portion (2.5-4.5 cm) is smaller in diameter than the rest of the tube. It is sized according to the ID of the tracheal portion. The shoulder (transition from oral to laryngotracheal portion) protects against inadvertent bronchial intubation. It cannot be used nasally as the larger segment will not pass through the nares. It is recommended for resuscitation but not long-term intubation.

Flexometallic Tube (Armoured/Reinforced/Spiral Embedded Tube) (Fig. 1.35)

These tubes have nylon or metal spiral reinforcing wire covered internally and externally by rubber, PVC or silicone. The spirals may not extend into proximal or distal ends. They are available in both cuffed and uncuffed forms.

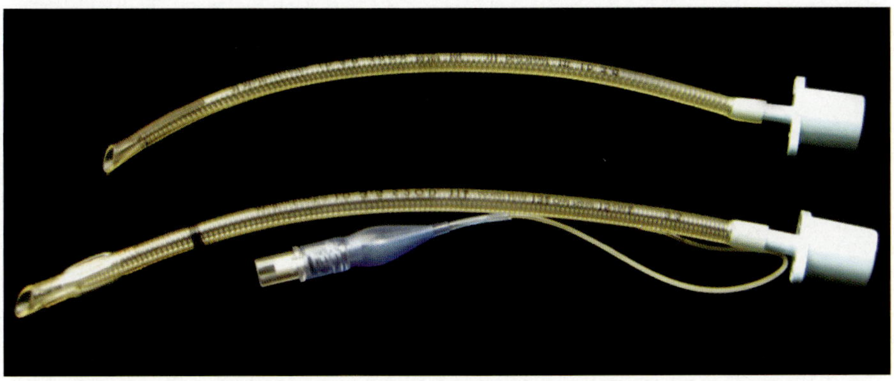

Fig. 1.35: Flexometallic endotracheal tube (cuffed and uncuffed)

Advantages
- Resistant to kinking or compression
- Portion of tube outside can be angled away from surgical field.

Disadvantages
- Requires a forceps or stylet for intubation
- Nasal insertion may be difficult
- Length cannot be shortened, so leads to increase in dead space
- Tendency to dislodge from secured position
- Not suitable for ventilation beyond operating room as once compressed due to teeth-bite, does not revert back to normal, so increases resistance to breathing
- Cuff deflation or failure of cuff to deflate.

Uses
- Prone position
- Head and neck surgery
- Surgery on trachea
- Patient with tracheostomy undergoing anesthesia.

Preformed Tube (Ring-Adair-Elwyn Tube/RAE Tube) (Figs 1.36A and B)

Both cuffed and uncuffed versions are available for oral or nasal use. As the diameter increases, the distance of the bend from distal tip also increases. There is a mark at the bend which should be at the teeth or nares when ideally positioned. Oral tubes (south pole tube) are shorter and have the bend at an acute angle so that it rests on patient's chin when positioned. A nasal preformed tube (north pole tube) has a curve opposite to oral tube; the outer portion is directed over the patient's forehead.

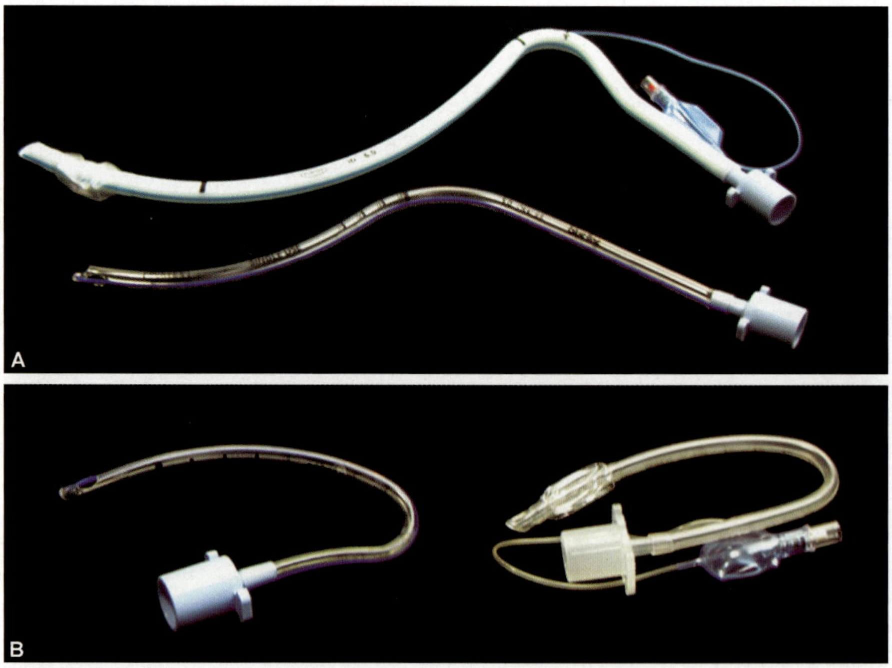

Figs 1.36A and B: Preformed tubes: (A) North pole tube; (B) South pole tube

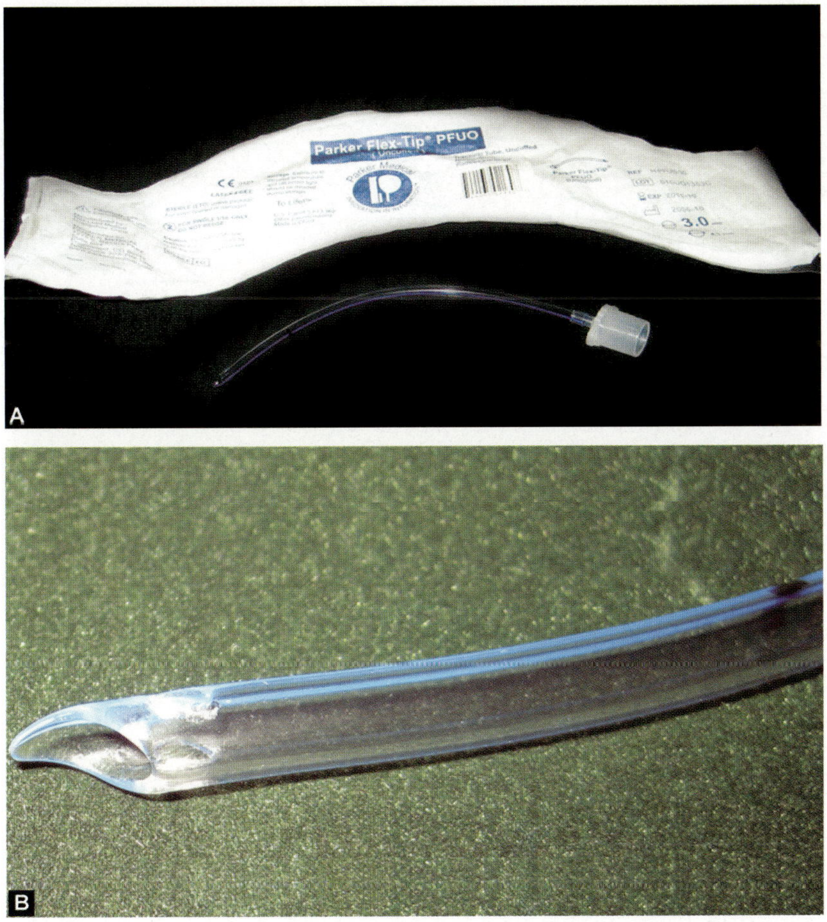

Figs 1.37A and B: (A) Parker flex-tip tube (3 mm ID); (B) Distal tip

Advantages
- Easy to secure and less chance of accidental extubation
- Breathing system connected away from surgical field.

Disadvantages
- Difficulty in passing suction catheter
- More resistance than conventional tube
- When inappropriately sized it may lead to bronchial intubation or accidental extubation.

Uses
- ENT surgery
- Dental surgery
- Plastic surgery.

Parker Flex-tip Tube (PFT Tube) (Figs 1.37A and B)

It has a "hooded" curved, flexible tapered tip that points towards the center of the distal lumen on the concave surface of the tube so that the bevel faces posteriorly. It reduces the gap between the fiberscope and inside of the tube. There are Murphy eyes on the right and left side of the tube. The tube cuff is very thin. The PFT tube is available in both cuffed and uncuffed version.

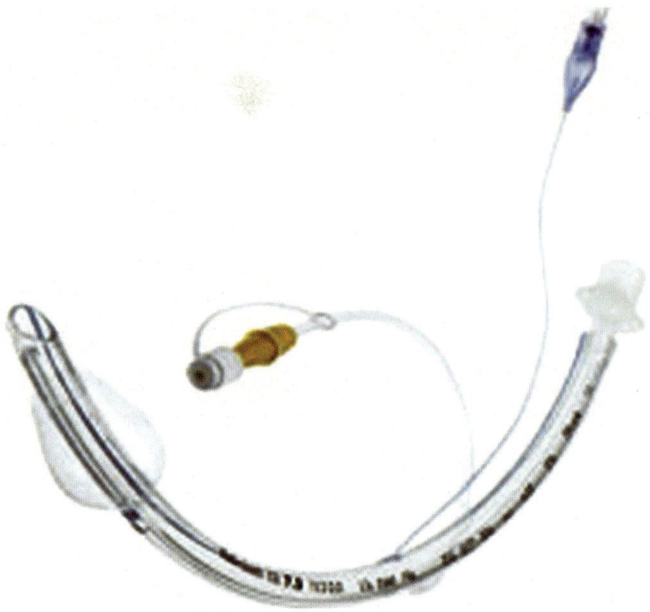

Fig. 1.38: Hi-Lo jet tracheal tube

Advantages
- Easier to advance over intubating guide or fiberscope
- Less likely to impinge on vocal cord.

Hi-Lo Jet Tracheal Tube (Fig. 1.38)

This specially designed tube has a main lumen for ventilation, an insufflation lumen integrated within the tube wall for delivery of jet ventilation and a distal monitoring/irrigation lumen used to monitor airway pressure, sample respiratory gases and irrigate the airway. It is used specifically for high frequency jet ventilation (HFJV) in neonatal/pediatric surgery.

The outer diameter of this tube is 0.8 mm larger than the conventional tube with same internal diameter. Thus, a 2.5 mm conventional tube has an outer diameter of 3.5 mm whereas the outer diameter of a similar triple lumen tube is 4.3 mm, which limits its use in infants weighing less than 900 gm. It is available in sizes starting from 3.0 mm onwards.

Table 1.12: Single lumen endotracheal tube

Internal diameter (mm)	*External diameter (mm)**
2.5	3.4
3	4.2
3.5	4.8
4	5.4
4.5	6.2
5	6.8
5.5	7.4
6	8.2
6.5	8.8
7	9.6

* cuffed tubes have approximately 0.5 mm additional outer diameter.

Options for One-Lung Ventilation

i. Single lumen ETT
ii. Bronchial blocker
iii. Double lumen tube (DLT).

Single lumen ETT: The conventional single lumen ETT is intentionally pushed into the right or left main bronchus. For left bronchus to be intubated, the bevel of ETT is rotated 180° and the head is turned to the right (Table 1.12).

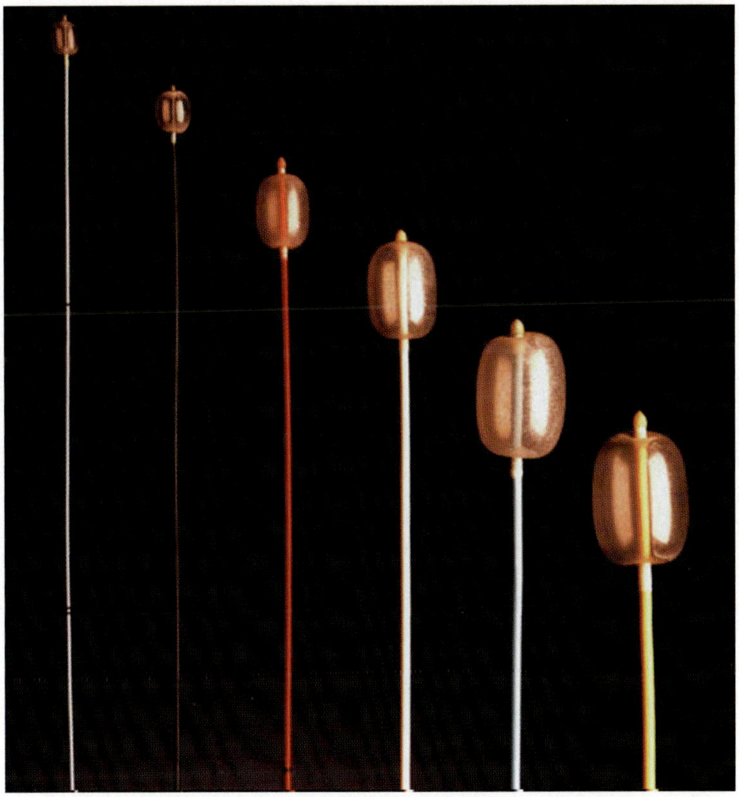

Fig. 1.39: Balloon-tipped embolectomy catheter

Advantages
- Simple, requires a fiberscope to confirm
- Preferred technique in airway hemorrhage or contralateral pneumothorax.

Disadvantages
- Failure to achieve adequate bronchial seal in case of uncuffed ETT leads to incomplete collapse of operated lung or failure to protect the healthy lung from contamination.
- Hypoxia from obstruction of upper lobe bronchus, when the right bronchus is intubated.

Bronchial blockers: Because many children are too small for DLTs, different bronchial blockers are often required for single-lung ventilation (SLV) in pediatric patients.

a. Balloon-tipped bronchial blockers **(Fig. 1.39)**
   1. Fogarty embolectomy catheter
   2. End-hole, balloon wedge catheter
b. Univent tube
c. Arndt bronchial blocker.

a. ***Balloon-tipped bronchial blockers***

1. *Fogarty embolectomy catheter:* Its placement is facilitated by bending the tip of the stylet towards the bronchus on the operative side. Fiberscope is used to confirm or reposition for appropriate placement.
2. *End-hole balloon wedge catheter:* The bronchus on the operative side is initially intubated with an ETT. A guidewire is advanced into that bronchus through the ETT. The ETT is then removed and the blocker catheter is advanced over the guidewire into the bronchus. The

Table 1.13: Balloon wedge catheters				
Size (F)	*Length (cm)*	*Maximum inflating volume (cc)*	*Inflated balloon diameter (mm)*	*Guidewire size (inches)*
5	60	0.75	8	0.025
6	60	1.0	10	0.035
7	110	1.25	11	0.038

ETT is reinserted into the trachea along the side of the blocker catheter. The catheter balloon is positioned in proximal mainstem bronchus under fiberoptic visual guidance **(Table 1.13)**.

Advantage of balloon-tipped blockers: More predictable lung collapse with optimal operating conditions is achieved than an ETT in bronchus.

Disadvantages

- Dislodgement of blocker balloon into trachea
- Being low-volume and high-pressure, overdistention can damage or rupture the airway
- With close tip bronchial blockers, operated lung cannot be suctioned and CPAP cannot be provided.

b. ***Univent tube:*** It consists of a conventional ETT with a second lumen containing a flexible small balloon-tipped tube which can be advanced into a bronchus to serve as a blocker. It requires a fibrescope for successful placement **(Table 1.14)** **(Fig. 1.40)**.

Advantages

- As bronchial blocker is firmly attached to main ETT, displacement is less likely than other blocker techniques
- High torque control blocker can block either left or right bronchus
- Easier to insert and position correctly than a DLT in difficult intubations because of its reduced bulk and anatomic angulation

Table 1.14: Univent tube		
Size-ID in mm	*OD (sagittal/ transverse) in mm*	*Age recommended (years)*
3.5	7.5/8.0	6–10
4.5	8.5/9.0	10–14
6	10.0/11.0	14–16
6.5	10.5/11.5	16–18

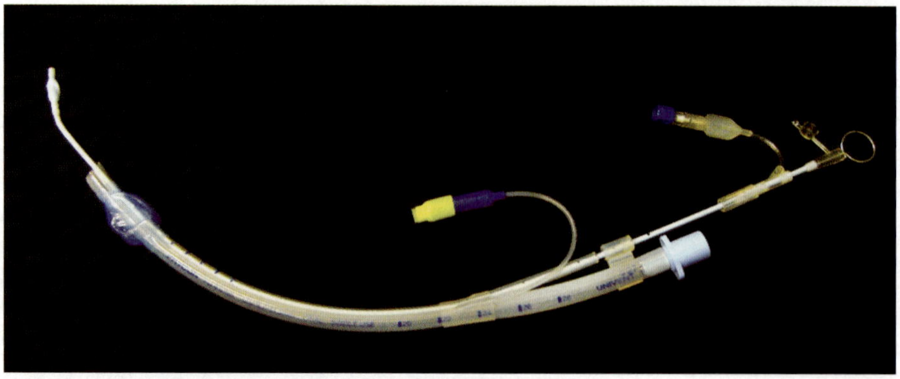

Fig. 1.40: Univent tube

- Can be used for postoperative ventilation
- Possible to use suction, apply CPAP, insufflate oxygen through blocker lumen.

Disadvantages
- Failure to achieve adequate bronchial seal
- Not recommended for children < 6 years of age
- Fixed shape causes difficulty in sliding over bronchoscope
- Does not soften in warm water bath
- Small lumen gets easily blocked by blood or pus
- Low volume high pressure cuff may cause mucosal injury
- Larger outer diameter makes it difficult to pass between cords.

c. ***Arndt bronchial blocker (wire-guided endobronchial blocker, WEB)* (Figs 1.41A and B):** It is designed to be used with a single lumen ETT already in place. It consists of two parts: a blocking catheter and a special airway (multiport) adapter. A 5F blocker can be inserted through ETT $\geq$ 4.5 mm ID. The innovative guide loop at the end of Arndt blocker's silicone balloon enables precise placement with a pediatric bronchoscope. Both bronchoscope and blocker can be introduced simultaneously through the multiport adapter while maintaining ventilation.

Advantages
- Can be used in already intubated or tracheostomized patients
- Has been used successfully in infants and small children

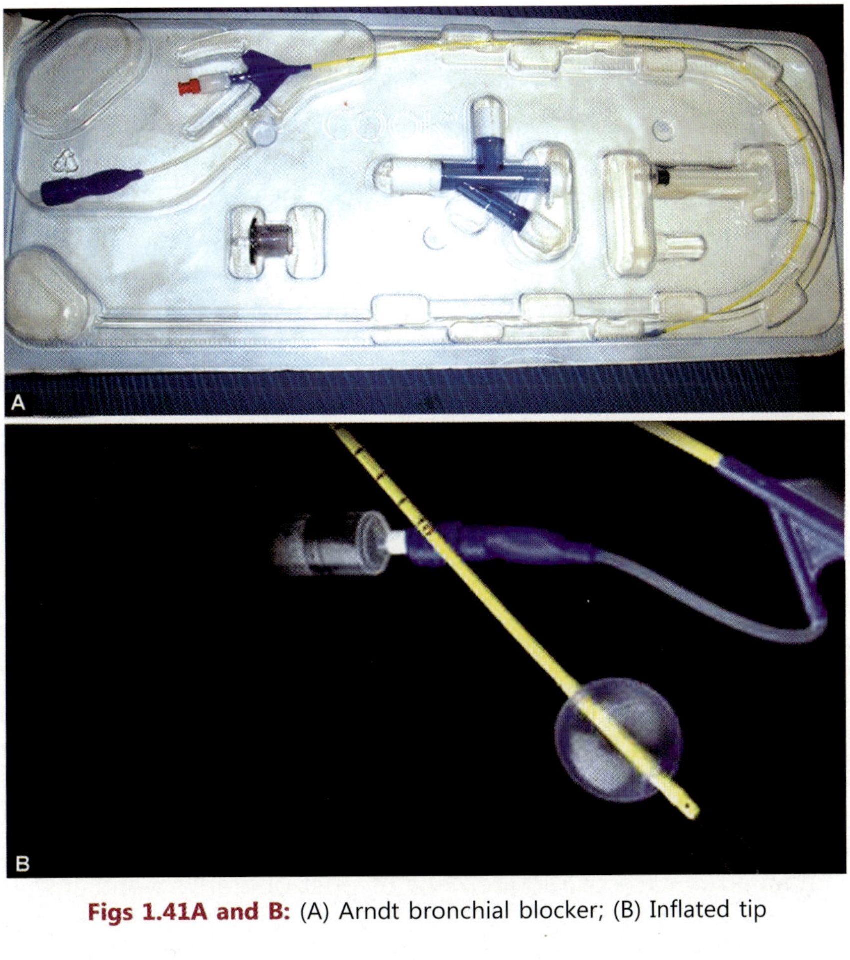

Figs 1.41A and B: (A) Arndt bronchial blocker; (B) Inflated tip

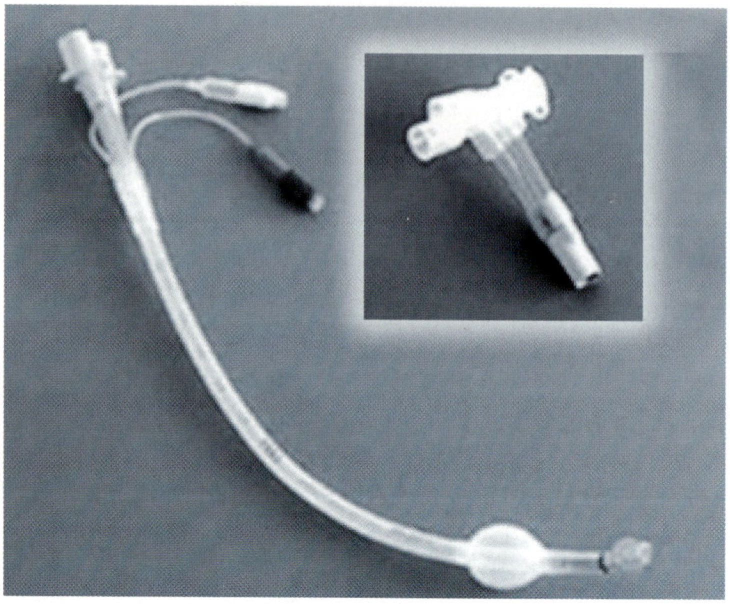

Fig. 1.42: Double lumen tube

- Allows larger internal cross-sectional area than a DLT or Univent tube of similar OD
- May require fewer insertion attempts than a DLT
- If the wire is removed, the lumen can be used for suctioning or administering oxygen or CPAP.

Disadvantages
- Once the wire loop is removed, it cannot be reinserted through the channel to allow repositioning of blocker
- Placement requires availability of fiberscope and skill to use it
- Takes longer to position and achieve complete lung collapse compared with Univent or DLT
- Balloon may get sheared while being removed from blocker port.

***Double-lumen tube (DLT)* (Fig. 1.42):** It consists of a shorter tracheal tube and a longer bronchial tube moulded together. Technique of insertion is the same as in an adult and requires a fiberscope to confirm placement. Left DLT is preferred to right DLT **(Table 1.15)**.

Table 1.15: Double Lumen tube

Size (F)	*Age (years)*	*Bronchial lumen OD (mm)*	*Main body OD (mm)*
26	8–10	5.1	9.3
28	10–12	6.9	10.2
32	12–14	8.1	11.2
35	14–16	9.7	13.5

Cuff thickness = 0.049 mm, therefore cuff adds to 0.1 mm to overall OD of the tube.

Advantages
- Ease of insertion
- Suction and CPAP with oxygen possible.

Disadvantages
- Often too large for small children
- Rigidity and width makes intubation difficult
- Tube malposition from head movement and surgical manipulation
- Trauma to the respiratory tract
- Needs to be changed in case of requirement of post-operative ventilatory support.

TRACHEOSTOMY TUBES (TT) (FIGS 1.43A TO C)

Various types of TT are available for intended use (Table 1.16).

- Cuffed, uncuffed or fenestrated
- Single cannula or double cannula
- Metal, plastic or silicone.

Plastic and silicone tubes are increasingly popular due to less weight and less crusting of secretions. Fenestrated tube has an opening that permits speech through the upper airway when the external opening is blocked. It is not recommended for small children as the opening can get obstructed with granulation tissue. The silicone tracheostomy tubes are available with air cuff or foam cuff and adjustable neck flange or extended connect.

Table 1.16: Neonatal and pediatric tracheostomy tube

Size	*ID (mm)*	*OD (mm)*	*Length (mm)*	
			Neonatal	*Pediatric*
3.0	3.0	4.5	30	39
3.5	3.5	5.2	32	40
4.0	4.0	5.9	34	41
4.5	4.5	6.5	36	42
5.0	5.0	7.1		44/50
5.5	5.0	7.7		46/52
6.0	6.0	8.3		54
6.5	6.5	9.0		56

Indications of Tracheostomy

- Congenital or acquired airway obstruction (i.e. Pierre Robin syndrome, subglottic stenosis, tracheomalacia)
- Long-term ventilation
- Neuromuscular diseases.

ALTERNATIVES TO CONVENTIONAL RIGID LARYNGOSCOPY IN CHILDREN

A. Gum elastic bougie aided endotracheal intubation
B. Lighted stylet aided endotracheal intubation
C. LMA/ILMA/LMA-C Trach aided endotracheal intubation
D. Indirect rigid fiberoptic laryngoscope assisted endotracheal intubation (i.e. Bullardoscope/Glidescope/Truview/C-MAC)
E. Flexible fiberoptic aided endotracheal intubation

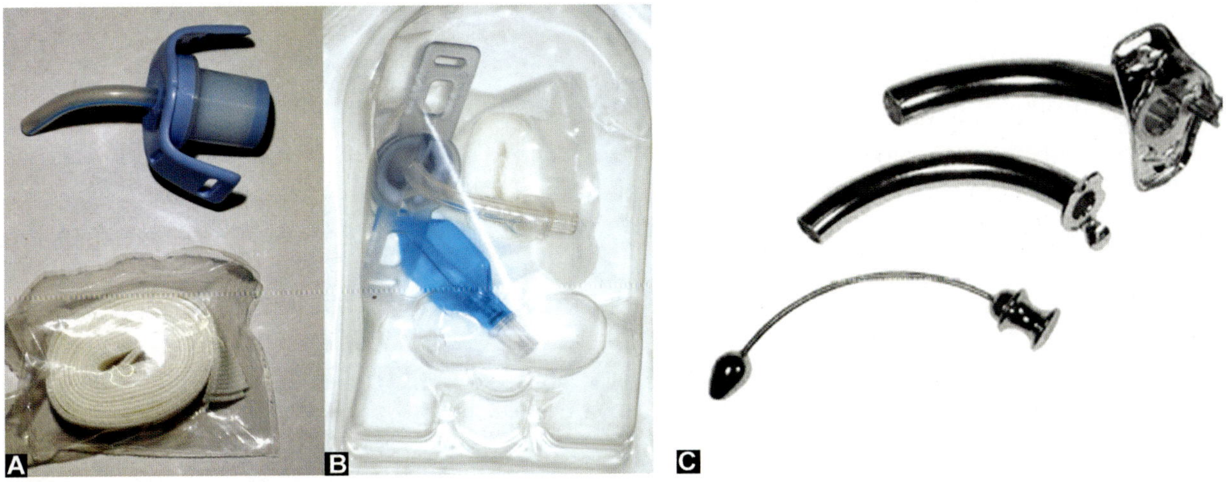

Figs 1.43A to C: (A) Neonatal tracheostomy tube; (B) Cuffed tracheostomy tube; (C) Metallic tracheostomy tube

F. Invasive airway access
    - Emergency needle cricothyrotomy
    - Transtracheal needle jet ventilation
    - Retrograde intubation
    - Tracheostomy

Endotracheal Tube Guides

A number of ETT guides including stylets, introducers and airway exchange catheters (AECs) have been used to aid intubation. The stylets and introducers are always an adjunct to direct laryngoscopy to provide directional control when the laryngeal inlet is not completely visible. A blind technique with these guides, even through the LMA, in difficult airway situations should be avoided **(Table 1.17)**.

Lighted Stylets

Depending on the structure and principle involved they can be broadly divided into two types **(Table 1.18)**:

a. Light wand (stylet with built-in light source): Functioning is based on transillumination of the soft tissues of the neck, does not require visualization of larynx, i.e. Trachlight
b. Intubating FO stylet (malleable stylet with built-in fiberscope and light source): based on visualization of larynx, i.e. SOS, FAST, etc.

Lighted stylets are portable, light-weight, easily cleaned and sterilized. They produce less sympathetic stimulation than direct laryngoscopy. The possible complications are minor airway trauma, arytenoid subluxation or instrument disarticulation that may be overcome by newer sturdier integral bulbs or FO bundle.

Trachlight

Indication: Difficult airway where fiberscope is unavailable or predicted to be difficult because of blood or secretions in the airway.

Contraindications
- Upper airway tumor or foreign body
- Retropharyngeal abscess
- Infection with friable tissue along intubation course
- Laryngeal injury
- Subglottic stenosis.

Caution: Transillumination may not be useful in emaciated or extremely obese children.

Technique: After lubricating the distal end of trachlight (TL) an ETT with a tube connector is loaded on. The tip of the stylet of TL should remain just inside the ETT without protrusion and locked with a clamp. The ETT-TL unit is shaped to 90°-120° "hockey-stick" at 3-6 cm from the distal end (i.e. just proximal to the cuff). The OR light is dimmed. In supine with head in neutral or sniffing position, perform jaw-lift and insert ETT-TL in midline to advance gently in a rocking motion. If resistance is felt, the TL is rotated backward, then the tip is redirected towards the thyroid prominence using the 'glow' as a guide. The initial well-circumscribed light just above the thyroid cartilage changes to a cone-shaped light projecting caudally at the suprasternal notch when it passes the vocal cords. Then the stylet is retracted 10 cm and the ETT-TL is advanced until the glow disappears at the sternal notch. Following the release of the locking clamp, the trachlight is removed from the ETT. In infants and small children, the

Table 1.17: ETT guides

S.No.	*Name*	*Description*	*Size /Length (cm) (OD)*	*Clinical applications*	*Special features*
1.	Stylet **(Fig. 1.44)**	Made of malleable aluminium, so adapts easily to desired shape. Its smooth high density polyethylene outer sleeve permits easy insertion and withdrawal	2.2 mm/22 5 4 mm/33.5, 67.3 5 mm/ 36.5, 69.3	for ETT (2.5–4.5 mm) for ETT (> 5 mm)	– Meant for single use only – Walking-stick design
2.	Eschmann tracheal introducer (Gum Elastic Bougie) **(Fig. 1.45)**	Made from a polyester woven base, angled 40° at its distal end (coude tip), calibrated at both ends at 10 cm increments for easy and accurate insertion. Marking indicate the direction of deflected tip	10 F/70 15 F/60, 70	ETT (4–5.0 mm) ETT (≥ 5.5 mm) Deflected tip should angle anteriorly to prevent posterior tracheal wall dissection by ETT during threading	– May cause trauma if excess force is applied or passed beyond carina – Both reusable and single use versions available
3.	Arndt airway exchange catheter (AEC)	Polyethylene, tapered end, multiple side ports, yellow in color, packaged with a stiff guidewire, bronchoscope port and Rapi-fit adapters	8 F/50 14 F/65, 78	ETT (3–5 mm) ETT (≥ 5.5 mm) – * Exchange of LMA and ETT using a fiberscope	– Single use – Allows both IPPV or jet ventilation
4.	Cook AEC **(Fig. 1.46)**	Polyethylene ID of catheter (mm) 1.6 2.3 3.0	8 F/45 11 F/83 14 F/83	ETT (≥ 3 mm) ETT (≥ 4 mm) ETT (≥ 5 mm)	
5.	Endotracheal tube guides	Straight, both single use and reusable versions available No hollow lumen or coude tip	5 F/50 10 F/70 15 F/70	ETT (≥ 2 mm)	5 F size available only for single use Used for exchange of ETT with a new ETT or speciality ETT in a known or suspected difficult airway.

* Fogarty catheter can be tried for its increased stiffness and its lumen allowing oxygen insufflation or jetted when smaller size AEC is not available.

Table 1.18: Lighted stylets

S.No.	Name / Manufacturer	Description	Sizes	Clinical application	Special features
1.	Trachlight **(Fig. 1.47)**	3 parts: a plastic reusable handle, a flexible wand with a bright bulb at distal end, a stiff retractable stylet. A proximal locking clamp secures ETT connector at the adjusted length	3 sizes: infant, child, adult Accommodates ETT $\geq$ 2.5-10 mm ID	– Fiberscope unavailable (ambulance or emergency dept.) – Fiberscopy difficult (Blood or secretions in airway) – War-time casualties	– Semi-blind technique – After 30 sec the bulb blinks off and on to prevent heat damage and also indicates 30 sec apnea time – Reusable 10 times
2.	Seeing optical stylet system (SOS) **(Fig. 1.48)**	High-resolution, stainless-steel, rigid FO stylet with preformed J-shape. Adjustable tube stop and integral oxygen port	Pediatric (ETT 3–5 mm) Adult (ETT $\geq$5.5 mm)	– Similar to flexible fiberscope – Comfortable for less experienced users with fiberscope	– Reusable – Simple form of a standard stylet with advantage of FO view and maneuverability of its tip. 6V Halogen battery or fiberscope light-source is required
3.	Flexible airway scope tool (FAST) **(Fig. 1.49)**	Similar to SOS, but has a malleable section and an atraumatic tip, easily adjusted manually to confirm patient's anatomy	Same as SOS	Same as SOS	– Recently modified to use nasally (FAST – Plus)
4.	Bonfils retromolar intubation fiberscope **(Fig. 1.50)**	High-resolution, rigid, FO stylet with fixed 40° curve distally. Adapter for fixation of ET and oxygen insufflation	Pediatric (2 mm) Adult (5 mm)	Similar to fiberscope Retromolar/transoral route – positions ETT directly in front of vocal cords with minimal manipulation of epiglottis	– Movable eyepiece allows ergonomic movement during intubation – Better maneuverability than flexible fiberscope – fast, atraumatic, reliable intubation in difficult airways
5.	Video-optical intubation stylet (VOIS) **(Fig. 1.51)**	Stylet malleable to 90° Angle of view 50°	Stylet diameter – 2.8 mm – 3.8 mm	Reliable and effective tool for management of difficult airway	– Used like a conventional stylet, but with a good view from the tip of tracheal tube – Needs least time and effort to learn

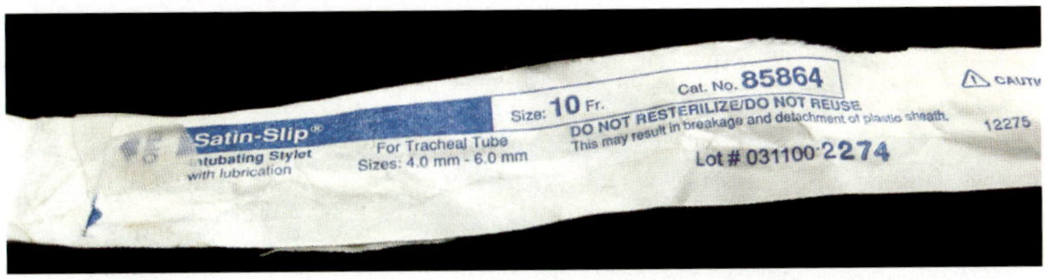

Fig. 1.44: Endotracheal tube stylet

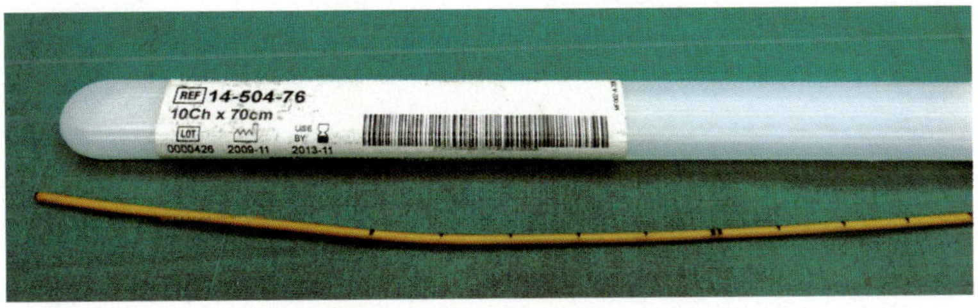

Fig. 1.45: Gum elastic bougie

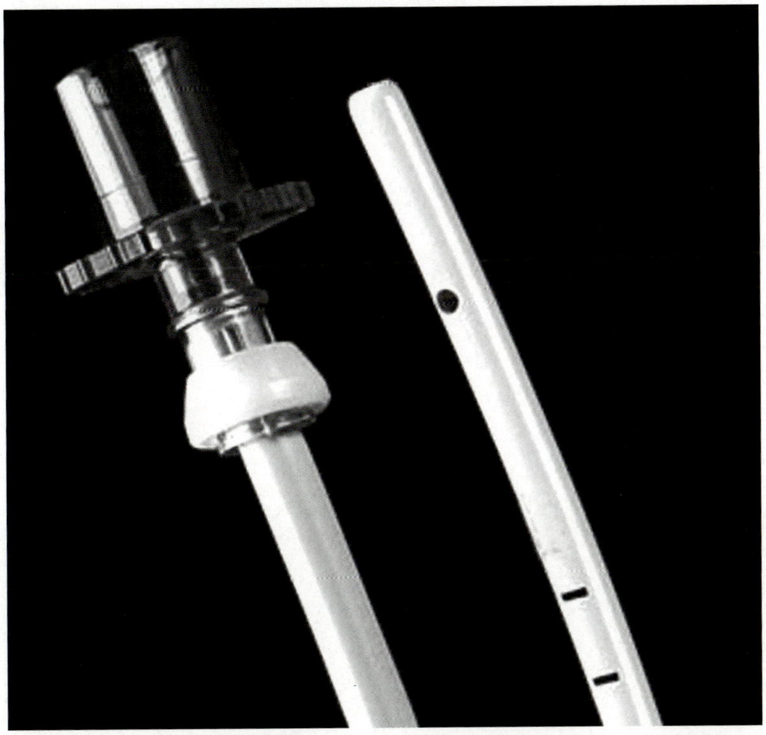

Fig. 1.46: Airway exchange catheter (cook)

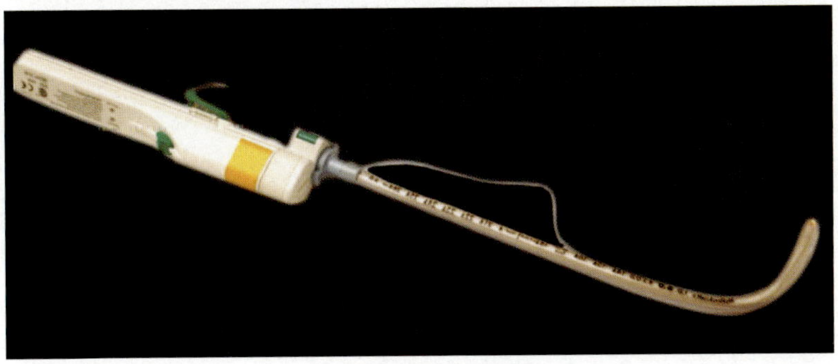

Fig. 1.47: Trachlight

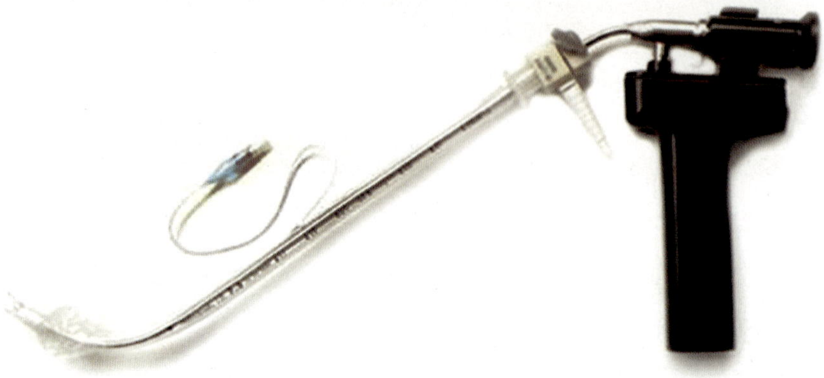

Fig. 1.48: Seeing optical stylet system (SOS)

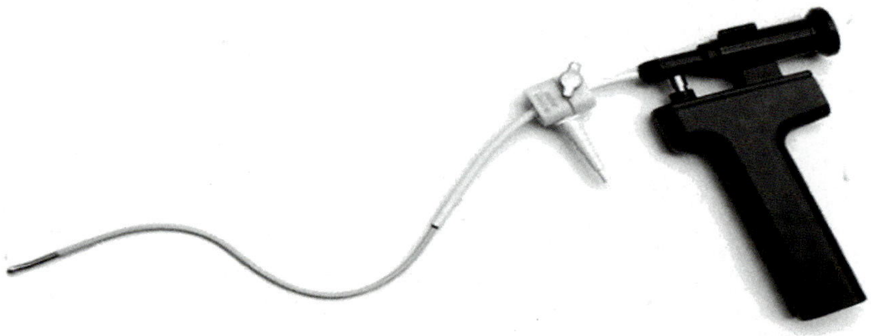

Fig. 1.49: Flexible airway scope tool (FAST)

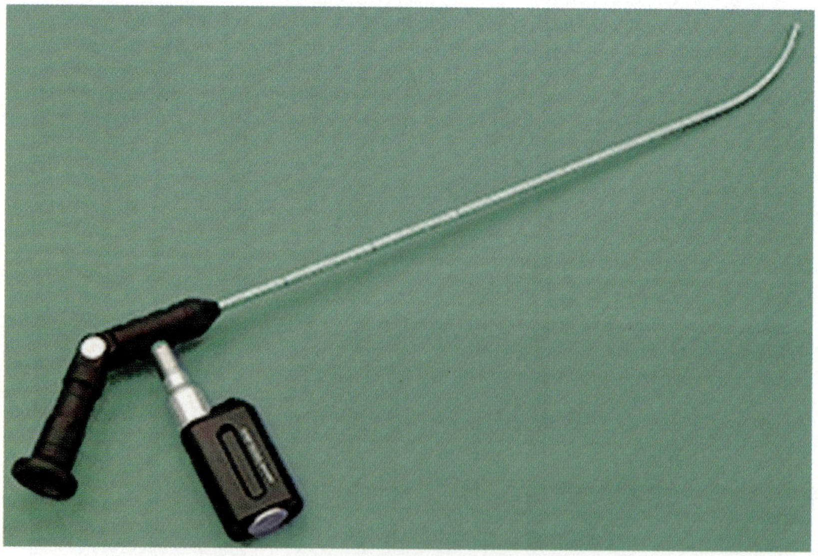

Fig. 1.50: Bonfils retromolar fiberscope

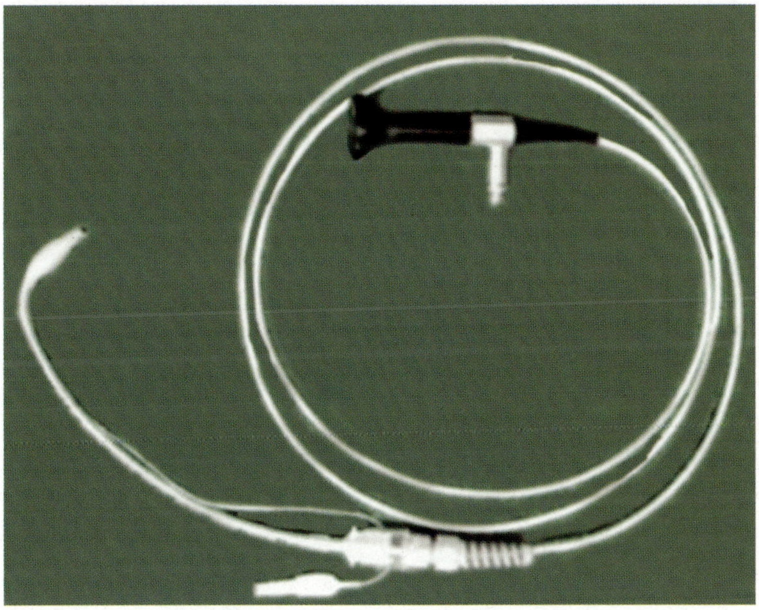

Fig. 1.51: Chhiber intubation fiberscope

feel of the lightwand is as important as the visual part. A click is often felt when the ETT/stylet is advanced past the epiglottis. It is easier to pass a slightly smaller ETT than the maximal age predicted diameter.

Laryngoscopes

A laryngoscope enables medical practitioners to approach the larynx, vocal cords, trachea and adjacent structures and provides a lighted view of the airway. Its use is primarily for inserting an endotracheal tube by intubating the trachea and also for examination of the throat to evaluate diseases of the larynx such as infection, congenital defects, growths, etc.

Laryngoscopy can be divided into: (a) Direct laryngoscopy, (b) Indirect laryngoscopy.

a. *Direct laryngoscopy:* It is a technique wherein the vocal cords are visualized using a handle with a detachable blade such as the Macintosh (curved) or the Miller (straight) blade. Choosing the correct size laryngoscope blade is critical to successful endotracheal intubation **(Table 1.19) (Figs 1.52A and B)**. The tip of Macintosh blade is placed in the vallecula and lifts the base of the tongue, thereby indirectly lifting the epiglottis for visualization of the vocal cords. The Miller blade directly lifts the epiglottis by being placed posterior to the epiglottis, so it is preferred in infants and younger children who have a large, floppy epiglottis **(Figs 1.53A and B)**. Excessive cricoid pressure should be avoided as it results in collapse of airway structures during intubation.

   The best conventional laryngoscopic view is dependent on the optimal positioning of the patient, an experienced practitioner with capable assistance for optimal external laryngeal manipulation (OELM) and backward upward right pressure (BURP) maneuver if required.

Table 1.19: Size of laryngoscope blade

Miller Blade		*Age Group*	*Macintosh Blade*	
Size	*Length (mm)*		*Size*	*Length (mm)*
00	65	Premature neonate		
0	75	Term neonate	0	80
1	102	Infant	1	87
2	155	Child	2	108

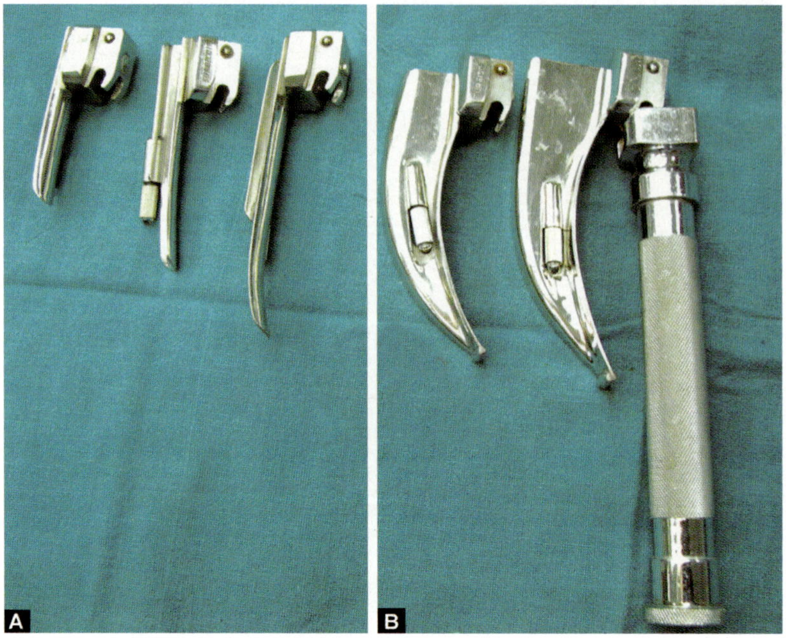

Figs 1.52A and B: Pediatric laryngoscope blade: (A) Miller blade (0, 1, 2) size; (B) Macintosh (1, 2) size

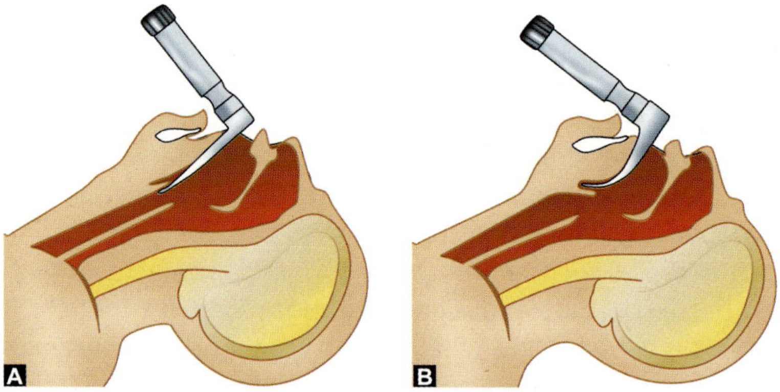

Figs 1.53A and B: Methods of laryngoscopy: (A) Miller blade; (B) Macintosh blade

b. *Indirect laryngoscopy:* The vocal cords are visualized through an optical or electronic imaging system. Modifications of the traditional laryngoscope blades are primarily designed for difficult airway situations such as limited mouth opening, anterior larynx, sternal space restriction, small intraoral cavity and unstable cervical spine. The most recently developed blades suitable for pediatric use are:
   i. Truview evo2
   ii. Glidescope
   iii. Bullard elite laryngoscope
   iv. C-MAC video laryngoscope
   v. Airtraq optical laryngoscope.

i. *Truview evo2* ***(Figs 1.54A and B)****:* This rigid, indirect laryngoscope has a unique blade tip angulation which provides a wide and magnified laryngeal view at 46° anterior refracted angle.

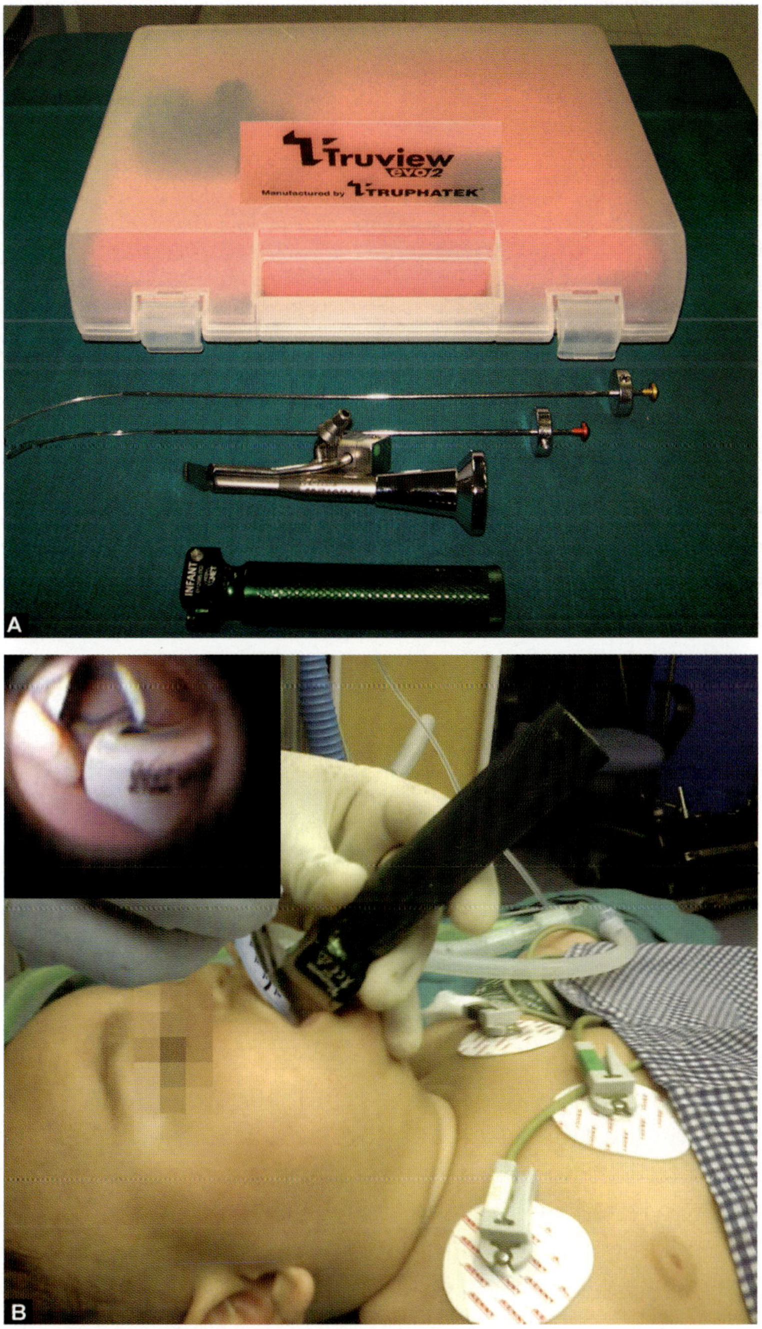

Figs 1.54A and B: (A) Truview evo2; (B) Truview in use

It has an integrated optical lens and an attachment for connecting oxygen (2-5 liters/min) which provides insufflation, prevents misting and improves safety. The narrow blade tip is suitable for a small mouth.

In the neutral position the laryngoscope is inserted centrally over the tongue or from the right side of the mouth, pushing the tongue to the left while visualizing through the optical eyepiece. First the uvula is seen, then the epiglottis becomes visible after advancing a little further. Here the blade can be used as MAC or Miller blade to lift the epiglottis and view the vocal cords. The endotracheal tube over the provided stylet is advanced along the side of the

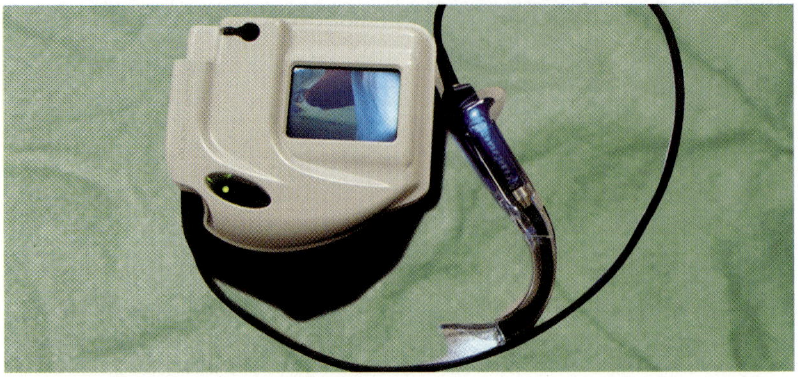

Fig. 1.55: Glidescope

blade till seen in the eyepiece. Then the ETT is advanced slightly upwards and to the left toward the tip of the blade to pass the cords. The ETT is further advanced into the trachea after removing the stylet.

Available in 2 sizes:
  i. Infant size (1-10 kg)
  ii. Adult size (>10 kg).

A new generation upgrade called Truview PCD is available in total 5 blade sizes out of which size 0, 1, 2 are for pediatric use.

Advantages
a. Effective in all intubation grades
b. Requires little or no neck movement
c. Reduced force required.

ii. *Glidescope* **(Fig. 1.55)**: This videolaryngoscope consists of a laryngoscope blade with a high-resolution digital camera in the middle of the tip of the blade and a LCD light source embedded along the inferior border. The blade is curved at 60° angle to match the anatomical alignment and the camera aids in video-assisted intubation by providing an outstanding view of the supraglottic area on the high-resolution display unit to the viewers. The overall thickness of the blade is reduced to 18 mm and it has an embedded anti-fogging mechanism. Midline approach is essential. A styletted ETT provides the needed curvature for insertion. It is available in 3 sizes—neonatal, pediatric and standard. The latest version called *Cobalt* uses a disposable blade and has an infant size with a smaller (10 mm) laryngoscope blade for use in neonates.

iii. *Bullard elite laryngoscope* **(Fig. 1.56)**: This indirect rigid fiberoptic laryngoscope combines the benefits of rigid direct laryngoscopy and fiberoptic intubation. It is available in three sizes – neonate - infant, child and adult. Its anatomically curved blade requires minimal mouth opening for insertion. Unlike in the adult Bullard, tip or blade extender is not used in children. Its power source can be a conventional laryngoscope blade with batteries and a halogen bulb or a fiberoptic light source attached through an adapter. It has a bifurcated channel: one working channel for oxygen insufflation, suction, instillation of local anesthetics or saline, passage of an airway exchange catheter or jet ventilation catheter and the other channel accepts the dedicated, non-malleable stylet.

Two stylets are available for use:
a. *Introducing (intubating) stylet:* It follows the blade contour to reach the field of vision at the 4 o'clock position. It facilitates the passage of the tracheal tube into the laryngeal inlet.

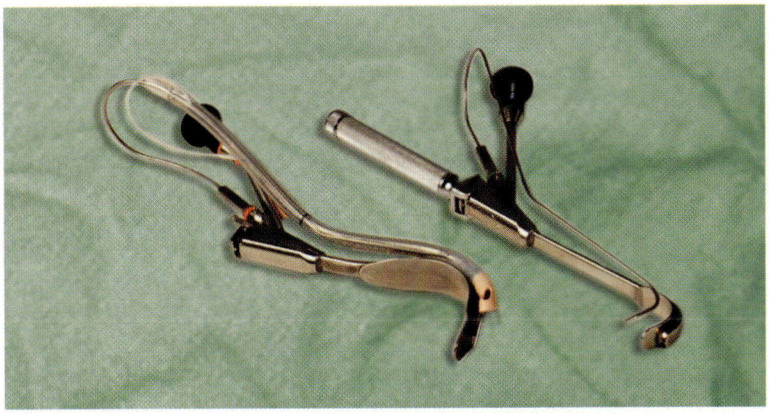

Fig. 1.56: Bullard elite laryngoscope

b. *Multifunctional stylet:* It is a long, hollow tube which follows the blade contour when attached. Its hollow core guides the flexible fiberoscope, tracheal tube exchanger or small catheter to instill local anesthetic into trachea. Its maneuverability is much less than the introducing stylet.

Its eyepiece is at 45° angle from the handle and can get attached to a video camera for remote viewing.

Recommendations for use: Six methods of intubation have been described. The blade-stylet assembly with premounted tracheal tube should be inserted into mouth in perfect midline over the tongue with the handle horizontal without looking through eyepiece. Then the handle is made vertical as it slides over the tongue to reach the pharynx. Here, for the first time the viewer has to look through the eyepiece to view the epiglottis and lift it directly or indirectly to slide the ETT over the introducer into the glottis.

Advantages
- Requires neutral head position
- Can be used for rapid sequence intubation in experienced hands
- Cheaper than fiberscopes, while indications are the same
- Quicker than flexible fiberoptic intubation
- Less trauma and discomfort in awake patient than direct laryngoscopy.

Disadvantages
- Requires skill and experience
- Expensive compared to conventional laryngoscope
- Takes slightly longer than conventional laryngoscopy
- Special tubes like DLT or laser tube cannot be inserted
- View less panoramic than regular intubation
- Not useful in distorted upper airway anatomy or foreign body obstruction or blood and secretions in the upper airway.

iv. *C-MAC video laryngoscope:* This video laryngoscope can be fitted with laryngoscope blades that are similar to Macintosh 1 or 2 blade and Miller 0 or 1 blade and are applicable in premature neonates **(Figs 1.57A and B)**. This unit is available with LCD monitor of 2.4" screen size which is movable via two rotation axes and rechargeable Li-ion batteries. It is light-weight, compact and very easy to use even by less-experienced practitioners.

v. *Airtraq optical laryngoscope:* Unlike other laryngoscope, it provides a channel for directing the ETT through the vocal cords. It is available in a variety of sizes, i.e. infants (gray),

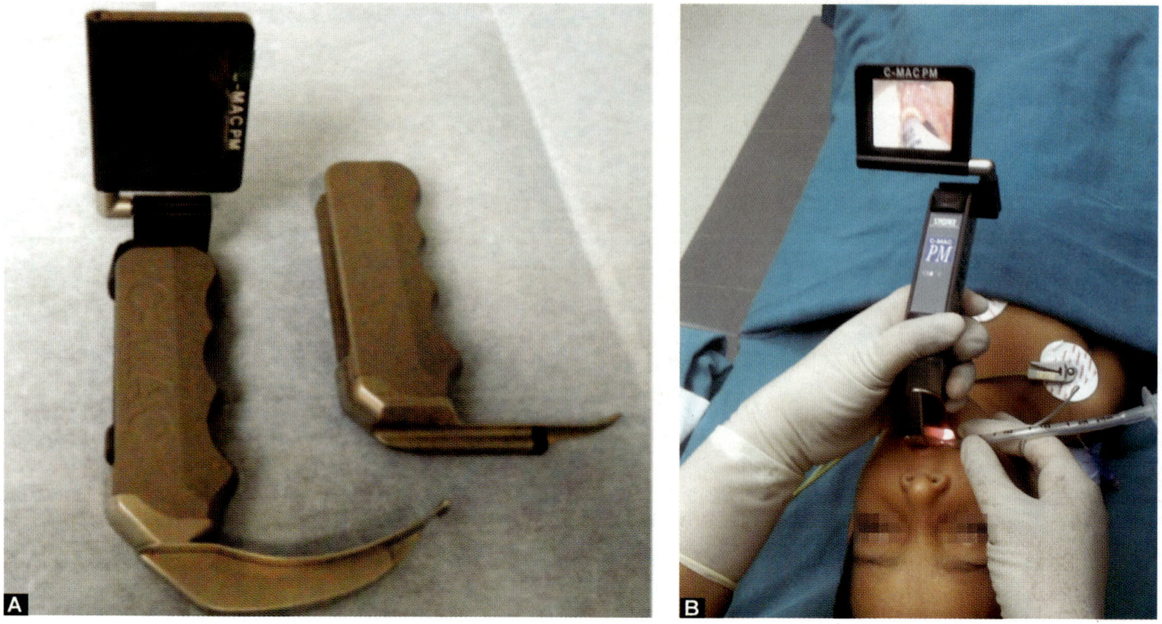

Figs 1.57A and B: (A) MAC 2 and Miller 1 blade; (B) C-MAC video-laryngoscope in use

pediatric (pink). The relatively large blade height (12-13 mm) precludes its use in infants with limited mouth opening.

Special Airway Techniques

A. Flexible fiberoptic intubation
B. Retrograde intubation
C. Cricothyrotomy
D. Tracheostomy.

FLEXIBLE FIBEROPTIC INTUBATION (FFI) (FIGS 1.58A AND B)

Flexible fiberoptic bronchoscopy remains the mainstay of airway assessment and difficult airway management. Indeed, it has become an integral part of neonatology, pediatric pulmonology, anesthesiology, critical care, laryngology and cardiothoracic surgery. The fiberscope is available in different sizes **(Table 1.20)**.

Advantages

1. It is less traumatic as it is manipulated under vision
2. It can be used orally or nasally for both upper and lower airway problems.

Table 1.20: Flexible fiberoptic bronchoscope

S. No.	*Type*	*Size (OD in mm)*	*LMA size/ ETT (ID in mm)*	*Indications*
1.	Neonatal (no suction port)	2.2	1 / 2.5	Premature neonates, infants
2.	Pediatric (most versatile)	2.9-3.1	2/3.5-4.5	Infant to 6-8 yr of age
3.	Adult	4-5.6	3 / ≥ 4.5	Older children and adolescents

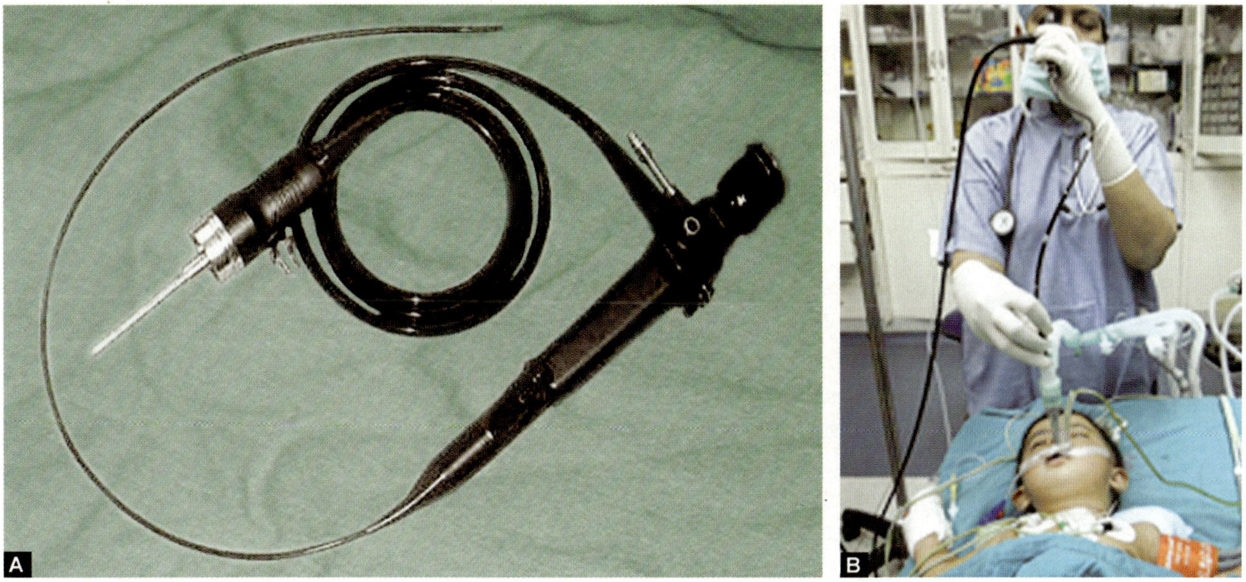

Figs 1.58A and B: (A) Flexible fiberoptic bronchoscope; (B) Fiberoscopy through PLMA

Disadvantages

1. It requires skill and experience
2. In case of abnormal anatomy, FFI may be impossible especially under deep sedation.

Indication

Diagnostic and treatment modality in airway management

Key-points for Procedure

1. The discrepancy between the OD of scope and ID of ETT should be kept to a minimum to prevent the ETT from getting stuck at the arytenoids while railroading over the scope.
2. For diagnostic bronchoscopy, the scope size should not be more than two-thirds of the diameter of the trachea as the patient has to breathe around the scope.
3. The neonatal fiberscope lacks a working channel which generates adequate suction. While using this scope secretions must be aspirated with a normal suction catheter. The neonatal fiberscope has very delicate ultra-thin optic fibers which get easily damaged and requires more skill to control.
4. During the oral approach in infants, the scope needs to make an acute anterior bend to approach the anteriorly placed laryngeal inlet, this problem is mitigated during nasal intubation.
5. The vocal cords in infants are slanted anteriorly, so it is ideal to approach the anterior commissure at the inlet and then make an acute posterior deflection to enter the trachea.
6. For FFI, the ETT is loaded on the scope before endoscopy and the tube is advanced after positioning the scope just above the carina and without having any slack on the scope.
7. If the child's trachea is too small for available scope, the suction channel of bronchoscope is used for passage of an extra-long J-tip guidewire into trachea under direct vision while the fiberscope sits above the vocal cords. The scope is then removed and the ETT can be advanced over the guidewire into the trachea. Alternatively, a stiffening device such as a ureteric dilator or Cooks airway exchange catheter can be railroaded over the guidewire. Next, the guidewire is removed and position of the catheter is confirmed by capnography.

Then an ETT can be railroaded over the stiffening device (However, the adult size fiberscope cannot be used in infants for railroading technique).

8. In case of any resistance during advancement of the ETT, it should be withdrawn and twisted 90° in counter-clockwise direction to make the tip free from the arytenoid cartilage. Reinforced ETT are preferable to minimize this problem.
9. Unlike in adults, an awake technique is not preferred in children since cooperation is required to gain a clear bronchoscopic view. A variety of regimens have been used for maintaining spontaneous ventilation in children undergoing FFI. Premedication with atropine helps to dry up secretions. Benzodiazepine with a relatively smaller dose of narcotic are preferred. Midazolam and remifentanil are the ideal agents for sedation as they are short acting and can be reversed with flumazenil and naloxone respectively. Ketamine and propofol are the most commonly recommended anesthetics, often supplemented with local anesthetic instillation and volatile anesthetics.
10. Nasal FFI is easier but nasal bleeding is a disadvantage and cannot be used in situations as cleft palate or adenotonsillectomy where oral intubation is required. Otherwise, the approach remains a personal preference.
11. Fiberscope through the LMA as a conduit and ventilation device is safe in neonates and infants.
12. Rescue techniques such as placing a retrograde guidewire through the suction channel may be employed if the glottis cannot be located with the scope or if blood and secretions are present. Once the fiberscope reaches the trachea, the ETT can be advanced. When the fiberscope is introduced through the LMA as a conduit, LMA has to be of split type or shortened or telescoping the tube over fiberscope is to be done to remove the scope and LMA. Telescoping involves pushing the tube of choice onto a larger one which acts as a holding device while removing LMA and scope without accidentally pulling out ETT.
13. FFI should be used early as an aid in a difficult airway scenario as presence of blood or secretions limit its use.

Contraindications

- Absolute – lack of time
- Relative – blood and secretions in oral cavity, edema of tongue, pharynx.

RETROGRADE INTUBATION

Retrograde intubation is an excellent technique for securing a difficult airway for both elective and emergency situations either alone or in conjunction with fiberscope and a tube exchanger. The technique is simple with a high success rate and should be a skill practiced by every anesthesiologist.

Indications

- Restricted cervical spine mobility
- Airway trauma.

Technique

Cricothyroid puncture is done with a small catheter-over-needle device with an attached syringe with cephalad angulation. A flexible J-tip guidewire (0.021 inch diameter, 140 cm) or an epidural catheter is introduced through the catheter to exit spontaneously through the mouth or nostril (in cases with difficult mouth opening, suction can be used to retrieve the retrograde catheter). The catheter at the cricothyroid membrane is removed and the guide is clamped at the skin.

The guidewire can be threaded through the ETT or AEC or working channel of a fiberscope sheathed with a reinforced ETT. The scope and tube assembly or AEC can be advanced following the wire through abnormal and collapsed tissues. Once the tip of the scope gets just below the vocal cords, the guidewire is removed with caudad traction. Then the scope is threaded into the distal trachea and ETT is slid into place. The airway exchange catheter will allow patient's oxygenation as well as confirmation of tracheal placement by capnography. The ETT can then be advanced over AEC.

Limitations

1. It may not be suitable for immediate intubation and ventilation as the procedure may take time for completion.
2. It may cause bleeding at the skin-puncture site, pretracheal abscess.
3. Trauma to the airway is possible, especially in infants, because of the poorly defined cricothyroid membrane and the proximity of the vocal cords to the puncture site.

CRICOTHYROTOMY

Cricothyrotomy is a life-saving procedure in CVCI situation. It can be performed by 3 techniques.

1. Needle cricothyrotomy
2. Percutaneous dilatational cricothyrotomy
3. Surgical cricothyrotomy.

Needle Cricothyrotomy

Needle cricothyrotomy with small catheters of at least 4 cm length with percutaneous translaryngeal ventilation (PTLV) is quicker, simpler and safer than the other two techniques. The jet ventilation catheter is available in 3 sizes (babies, children and adults). Catheter length is important, because if too short, it may come out and gas will escape into the subcutaneous tissue of the neck. It is essential for every emergency physician to be familiar with the indications, contraindications, techniques and complications of this type of rescue airway.

Indications: "CVCI situation"

- Facial or cervical trauma, uncontrollable oral hemorrhage
- Oropharyngeal edema from infection, anaphylaxis or chemical inhalation injuries.
- Trismus or anatomic variants
- Rescue from profound hypoxemia during FFI under deep sedation, followed by urgent tracheostomy.

Contraindications

- Where nasal or oral intubation possible and safe
- Acute laryngeal trauma or infection
- Obstruction at or below the cricoid level, as the obstructing element may get pushed deeper
- Avoided if patient recently intubated
- Inability to locate the cricothyroid membrane
- Upper airway obstruction not allowing the gas to escape.

Technique

- Identify the cricothyroid membrane in the midline between thyroid and cricoid cartilage. Prepare skin with betadine.
- Use a small 25 G needle with syringe to aspirate air through the cricothyroid membrane and inject 0.3 ml lignocaine (2%) transtracheally.

- Next use a large 12-14 G angiocath (catheter over needle) with syringe directed at a 45° angle caudally to puncture the membrane.
- Once air is aspirated into the syringe, remove the needle from angiocath while advancing the catheter smoothly in a caudad direction, taking care not to perforate the posterior tracheal wall.
- Confirm the position of the catheter by air aspiration with a syringe.
- Then attach the catheter hub to an oxygen source or jet ventilator through an appropriate connector.

This technique is a temporary measure which allows 30-40 minutes of uninterrupted oxygenation and ventilation while allowing unhurried access to secure the airway. Significant barotrauma is a risk with tracheal jet insufflation. A high-flow oxygen source and an adequate expiratory time are the appropriate ventilatory parameters to limit barotrauma.

Complications
- Exsanguinating hematoma
- CO_2 retention in spite of adequate oxygenation
- Perforation of esophagus, posterior wall of trachea, thyroid gland
- Inadequate oxygenation
- Subcutaneous or mediastinal emphysema
- Infection.

Percutaneous Dilatational Cricothyrotomy (PDC)

This technique uses the Seldinger method to gain access to the cricothyroid membrane. The track around the guidewire can be enlarged by using serial dilators to accommodate the cricothyrotomy tube which may have a cuff. There are a number of commercial kits available. For example, Quicktrach 2 mm for children, Arndt emergency cricothyrotomy cath set (9F/6 cm length, coil reinforced kink- resistant catheter with a standard 15 mm connector and luer-lock) **(Fig. 1.59)**.

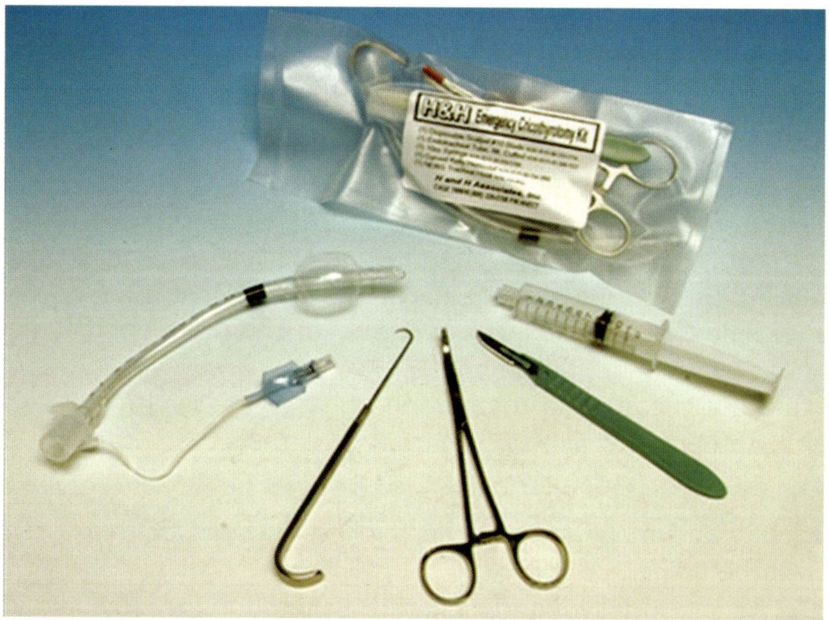

Fig. 1.59: Percutaneous dilatational cricothyrotomy set

Surgical Cricothyrotomy

In this technique a transverse incision is made through the cricothyroid membrane using a scalpel, through which an ETT is inserted. It should be performed rapidly when equipment for less invasive technique is unavailable. It is a more definitive airway than the PDC.

TRACHEOSTOMY

Tracheostomy may be defined as establishing transcutaneous access to the trachea below the level of cricoid cartilage.

Indications

1. Emergent—acute airway loss in <6 yr of age where the cricothyroid space is too small for cannulation
2. Elective—distorted laryngeal anatomy, prolonged ventilatory support.

Percutaneous dilatational tracheostomy is not recommended in the pediatric age group as the tracheal tissue is markedly elastic in children. Pressure applied on the anterior tracheal wall during dilatation of stoma can cause compressive obstruction of tracheal lumen and increased chance of perforation of the posterior wall of the trachea.

Translaryngeal tracheostomy is preferable in children as its approach is retrograde and requires minimum pressure on the pretracheal tissue and trachea. Under bronchoscopic guidance, insertion of a J-shaped wire percutaneously in the trachea passes retrograde into the mouth. The specially designed conal dilator with tracheostomy tube is threaded over the guidewire and pulled through the oral cavity, larynx, trachea and out through the anterior tracheal wall. Then the cone is removed and TT is rotated from a cephalad to caudal direction by using an obturator and then advanced caudally to its final position. During the procedure, the trachea is ventilated with a small diameter tracheal tube positioned co-axial to the original airway and its distal end is positioned distal to tracheostomy site. The ETT is removed after or just before rotation and securing of tracheostomy tube. Since dilatation is achieved by tracheal cannula itself (tracheal rings are simply divaricated), it fits snugly with the wound edges. This newer technique is safe in children and specially beneficial in coagulopathic babies.

The subcricoid region has the advantage of absence of bleeding as no major blood vessel is present on the cricotracheal membrane and also reduction in possible development of subglottic edema and stenosis.

Surgical tracheostomy is more invasive. In the supine position, maximal extension of the head and neck is done with a towel roll. A 1 cm transverse skin incision is made in the second tracheal ring. The incision is dilated and deepened. A longitudinal tracheal incision is made over the second and third tracheal ring and a tracheostomy tube is inserted through the opening. The tracheal cartilage should not be excised as this leads to stricture formation. A metal tube is avoided. Ideally intubation should be done prior to tracheostomy unless an obstructive lesion precludes its use. Sedation and analgesia is strongly recommended to minimize movement of the head and neck for 3-5 days.

Difficult Airway

Management of a difficult airway is a fundamental part of clinical practice. Fortunately, the incidence of unexpected difficult pediatric airway is low since most of them are associated with congenital syndromes.

Recognizing a difficult airway is thus the first step in handling these cases. A detailed preoperative evaluation and accordingly a plan of action of how to proceed with the available resources and equipment, usually prevents a CVCI situation. A child's airway anatomy may get modified with growth or get worsened in some syndromes, thus a previous successful intubation does not guarantee success in the future. Airway assessment is very difficult in an uncooperative child. Every child's airway should be evaluated in the lateral profile. A full and frank discussion of the risks with parents (and child if appropriate) and the possibility of tracheostomy and indeed, of failure to secure the airway should always be mentioned.

Preparing these patients is the next step. Premedication and duration of preoperative fasting plays an important role in preventing a crying child, as upper airway obstruction worsens when the child cries or struggles and generates a greater negative intrathoracic pressure. Premedication with atropine is recommended, to dry up secretions and to prevent bradycardia associated with airway manipulation.

COMMON CAUSES OF DIFFICULT AIRWAY

- Congenital craniofacial abnormalities
  a. Maxillary hypoplasia: Apert syndrome, Crouzon disease
  b. Mandibular hypoplasia (micrognathia): Pierre-Robin syndrome, Treacher-Collins syndrome, Goldenhar syndrome, Nager syndrome
  c. Mandibular hyperplasia: Acromegaly, Cherubism
- Temporomandibular joint ankylosis: Congenital, mucopolysaccharidoses (MPS)
- Microstomia: Ludwig's angina, burns, trauma scarring, hemangioma tongue, Freeman-Sheldon syndrome.
- Macroglossia: Down's syndrome, hypothyroidism, MPS, Beckwith-Wiedeman syndrome
- Nose: Narrow nares due to MPS, choanal atresia
- Pharynx: Hypertrophic tonsils and adenoids, retropharyngeal abscess
- Palate: Cleft palate, soft palatal swelling
- Larynx: Glottic-laryngomalacia, MPS,
  Infraglottic- congenital stenosis, MPS
- Neck-vertebral anomalies: MPS, Klippel-Feil anomaly.

Any of the above can lead to a difficult airway due to:

a. Difficult access, i.e. limited mouth opening, obstruction by soft tissue mass
b. Difficult to visualize, i.e. small mandible with less submandibular space to accommodate tongue.
c. Challenges on target tissue, i.e. inspite of glottic visualization, unable to ventilate or intubate as in foreign body trachea or laryngeal tumor.

MANAGEMENT STRATEGIES (FIG. 1.60)

The principles of airway care in the adult population are applicable to pediatric patients. However, the techniques available in adult care may not be available because of size and technological limitations.

1. The degree of cooperation in the pediatric age group is variable, so awake intervention may not always be an option.
2. Loss of patency of child's airway rapidly results in hypoxemia and desaturation due to a low FRC with a high basal oxygen consumption. Oxygen supplementation throughout the intervention is critical in children.

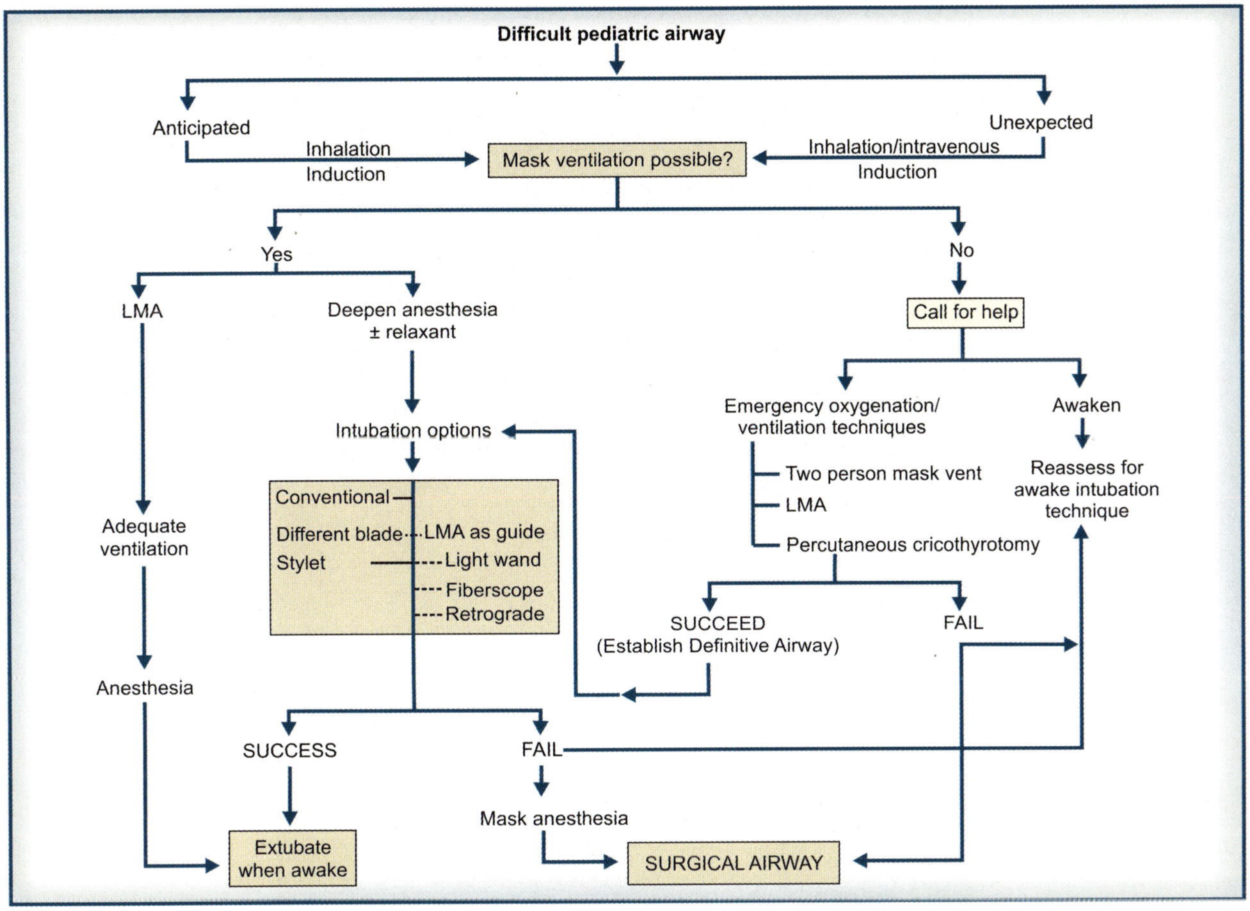

Fig. 1.60: Difficult pediatric airway algorithm

3. In certain cases, mask ventilation is difficult but airway access via LMA or ETT is achieved readily. In such situations, an attempt with LMA insertion or tracheal intubation should be a prudent first intervention.
4. A patent airway is the ultimate goal, hence direct laryngoscopy attempts must not be persistent because of associated morbidity and mortality and other choices should be offered as an alternative according to algorithm.
5. Transtracheal techniques should be considered early if alternate transoral techniques are either not available or do not achieve ventilation.
6. Maintenance of spontaneous breathing allows a way out in case of inability to secure the airway. Muscle relaxants should be withheld until the airway is secure and intubation should be preferably be done under deep inhalation anesthesia. In case muscle relaxant has led to a "CVCI" situation, surgical airway should be rapidly accessed.
7. For the neonatal difficult airway, the presence of a third competent person is advisable. When bag and mask ventilation, LMA and tracheal intubation all fail to establish effective ventilation, the possibility of a laryngotracheal anomaly calls for an immediate surgical access as the only way to save the baby.
8. Planned extubation of a trachea that presented difficulty at intubation, should take place in the presence of not only an experienced laryngoscopist but also a surgeon competent in providing surgical access to the airway.

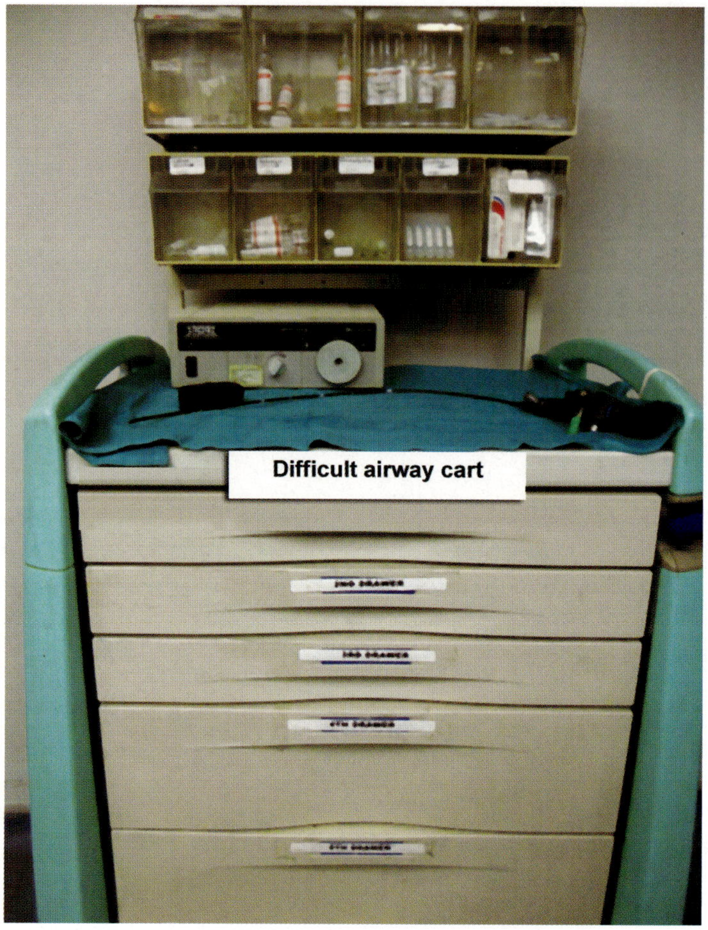

Fig. 1.61: Difficult airway cart

DIFFICULT AIRWAY CART FOR PEDIATRICS (FIG. 1.61)

One should ideally have all the desired equipment on a designated difficult airway cart. However, it is far more important that the kit contains tools with which the physician is familiar and skilled, than containing a large number of items. All equipment should be clearly labeled and functionally well-maintained.

A Standard Airway Kit

A Standard airway kit should contain as a minimum:

- Face-masks of all sizes and shapes
- Nasopharyngeal airways and oropharyngeal airways- of all sizes
- ETT - uncuffed and cuffed (2.5-6 mm)
- Tracheal tube stylet (6F, 8F)
- Magill forceps—small, medium
- Laryngoscope blades - Miller (00, 0,1,2), Macintosh (0,1,2), short laryngoscope handle
- LMA classic (1,1.5,2,2.5,3), ProSeal (1, 1.5,2,2.5, 3) disposable LMA
- Suction catheters (6F, 8F, 10F, 12F) **(Fig. 1.62)**
- Manual resuscitation bag (0.5L and 1 Liter)
- Miscellaneous—spare batteries, lignocaine spray, lubricant, bite-block, syringes, decongestant.

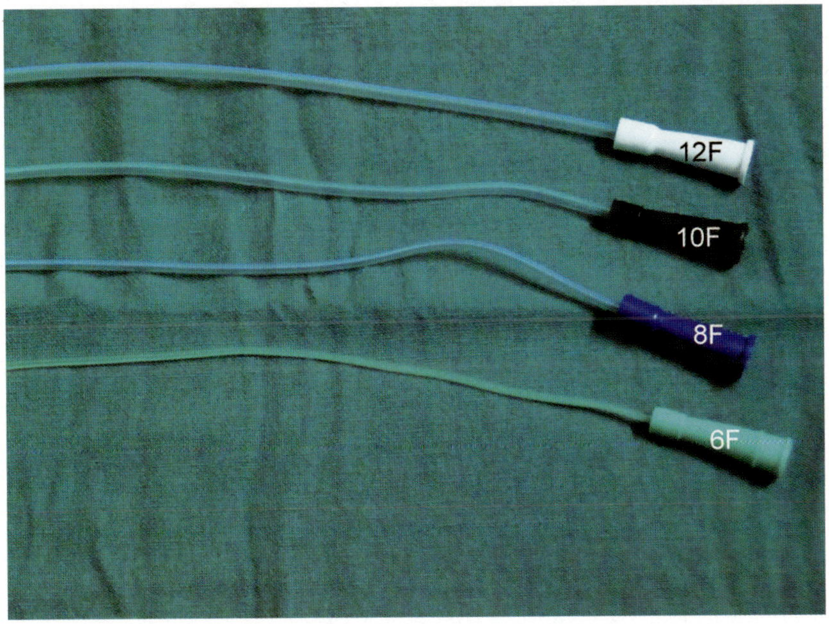

Fig. 1.62: Color coded suction catheters

A Difficult Airway Cart

A difficult airway cart should contain:

- Lighted stylet (Trachlight) - Pediatric and infant size
- Gum elastic bougie (GEB)
- Airway exchange catheter (AEC)
- Alternative to direct laryngoscope
  - Flexible fiberscope
  - C-MAC video laryngoscope
  - Retromolarscope

  } Pediatric size
- Transtracheal airway kit - l6/18G IV catheter (1.5-2 inches long jet ventilation device)
- Cricothyrotomy equipment
- Tracheostomy set
- Oxygen source
- ILMA # 3, Combitube (37F).

2 Vascular Access

This chapter on vascular access comprises of three sub-headings:
1. Venous access
2. Arterial cannulation
3. Intraosseous access

Venous Access

Venous access can be broadly categorized as:
A. Peripheral venous access
B. Central venous access.

PERIPHERAL VENOUS ACCESS

It is the method of choice of vascular access in most non-emergent situations. Venous cannulae are available in a variety of sizes (26G, 24G, 22G, 20G) **(Fig. 2.1)**.

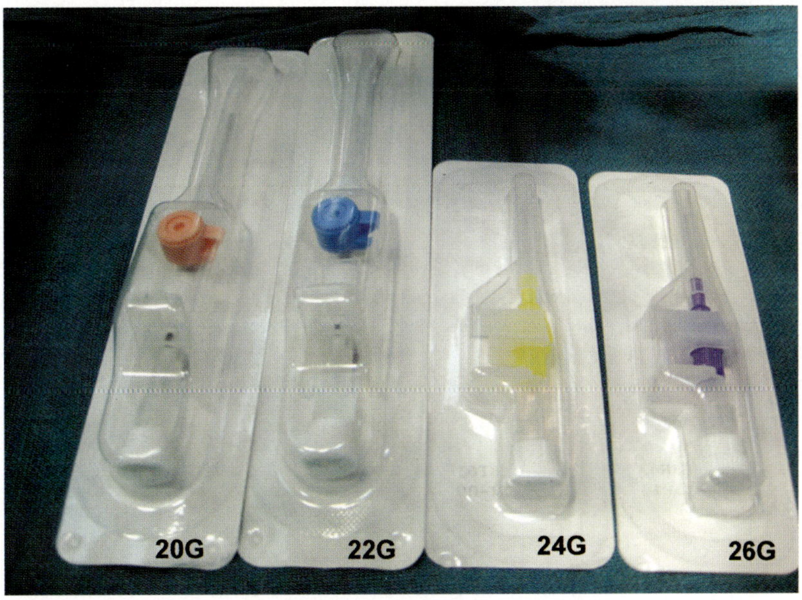

Fig. 2.1: Intravenous cannulae

Indications

1. Administration of drugs and intravenous fluids
2. Blood sampling.

The veins of the dorsum of the hand should be the first choice. Others such as cephalic, basilic and median antecubital veins are relatively large and therefore easy to cannulate, but they should be reserved as second choices in case a peripherally inserted central catheter (PICC) or venous cutdown is required.

Special considerations in neonates:

- Conserve sites to preserve limited venous access: use distal sites first
- Use IV cannula 24G–22G for sampling as hemolysis may occur with 25G or smaller needles
- Veins on the dorsum of feet and superficial scalp veins (frontal, superficial temporal, posterior auricular and occipital veins) are convenient access points in neonates.

Technique

Aseptic precautions should be followed. Occlude vein proximally using finger compression for neonates or tourniquet for older children **(Figs 2.2A and B)**. The tourniquet should be inflated

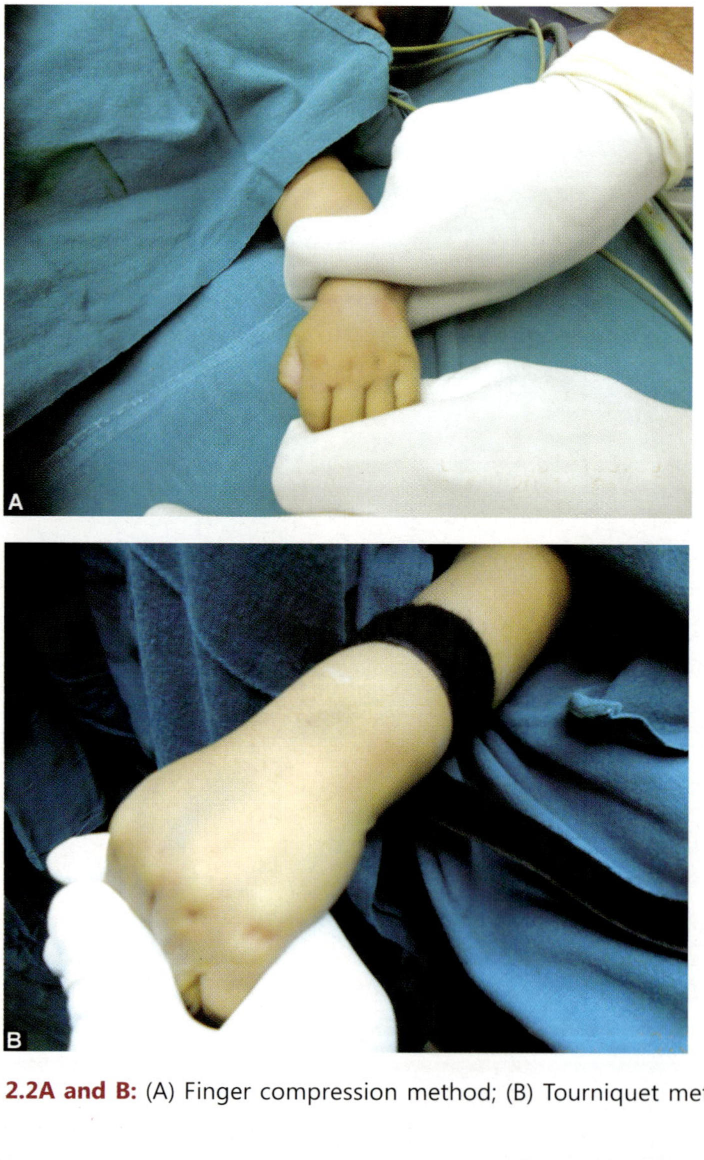

Figs 2.2A and B: (A) Finger compression method; (B) Tourniquet method

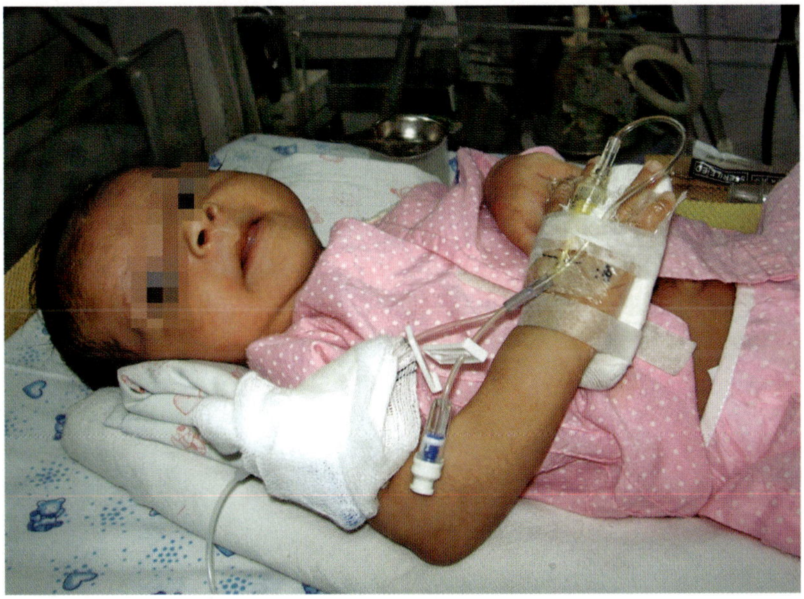

Fig. 2.3: 24G IV cannula *in situ*

to a pressure between systolic and diastolic blood pressure to ensure arterial flow to the limb. Penetrate skin first a few millimeters distal to the point of entry into the vessel and then introduce the needle into the vessel until blood flashback appears in the cannula. Angle of entry should be 25°–45°. Bevel should face upward for optimal blood flow, however, during shock aiming the bevel down may facilitate entry into constricted vein. Advance the outer cannula while keeping the puncture needle in place. Release the tourniquet or occlusion.

A "flash back" of blood into the catheter tubing may not occur in very small babies. In such a case, the catheter should be flushed with normal saline to confirm its proper placement. Improper placement leads to swelling of surrounding tissue. Adequate stabilization should be used to prevent its dislodgement **(Fig. 2.3)**. It is preferable initially to cannulate a small visible vein on the hand or foot after inhalational induction and subsequently change to a larger bore needle, if required. For treatment of compensated shock, a large bore peripheral catheter is ideal to enable rapid delivery of a large volume of fluid.

Merits
- Ease of insertion
- Low cost
- Minimal complications.

Demerits
- Easily blocked or dislodged
- Potential for local tissue injury
- Hematoma, thrombosis, phlebitis, cellulitis
- Embolization of formed clot with vigorous flushing
- Air embolism
- Suitable only for small-to-moderate infusion volumes
- Not suitable for hypertonic solutions or irritant drugs.

CENTRAL VENOUS ACCESS

For central venous access, a major difference between children and adults is that in pediatric patients, the age and particularly weight and length of the patient are decisive factors determining the choice of central venous catheter (CVC) type and caliber. Percutaneous insertion of CVCs can be achieved through venipuncture or via surgical method. Percutaneously inserted non-tunnelled CVCs are used for a short to intermediate indwelling period, whereas tunnelled catheters are used for a longer indwelling period (weeks or months). In older children it may be inserted under sedation and local anesthesia, but small children often require general anesthesia for subclavian and jugular access. The incidence of complications associated with CVC insertion may be low, but the consequences may be severe. Knowledge of anatomic landmarks is essential for CVC placement. Whenever possible, ultrasound should be used to identify the course of vessels, particularly in difficult anatomy or suspected thrombosis of vein.

Indications for Central Venous Access

- Total parenteral nutrition
- Chemotherapy
- Emergency access (trauma, CPR)
- Critical care monitoring (CVP, PCWP)
- Vasoactive drug therapy
- Long-term antibiotics (>3-4 weeks)
- Frequent sampling and medication in chronically ill children
- Fluid management.

Contraindications

- Infection or burn over insertion site
- Uncorrected coagulopathy
- Venous thrombosis of the vessel
- Lack of parental consent in non-emergency setting.

Choice of Veins

- Internal jugular vein
- Subclavian vein
- External jugular vein
- Femoral vein
- Antecubital vein
- Umbilical vein.

The length of CVC should be determined according to the size of the patient and entry site of catheter **(Fig. 2.4)** **(Table 2.1)**. Introducing needle and catheter gauge should be closely matched to reduce blood loss from the insertion site. Risk for CVC induced thrombosis increases with increased ratio of catheter to vessel size, longer indwelling time, parenteral nutrition and malignancy. Polyurethane or polyethylene material is preferable to silicone rubber because of the following reasons:

- More durable and biocompatible
- Stronger and higher tensile strength

- Thermosensitive, soften once inserted
- Smoother, so minimize protein and platelet adhesions, reduce fibrin and thrombin formation
- Radiopaque.

INTERNAL JUGULAR VEIN CANNULATION

Internal jugular vein (IJV) is the preferred site for percutaneous CVC access when short indwelling time (<5 days) is expected. Right IJV is preferable to left as there is less risk of pneumothorax and thoracic duct injury and greater chance of passing into the SVC instead of right subclavian vein (i.e. shorter and more direct route to SVC).

Table 2.1: Different sizes of central venous catheters

Needle size (G)	*Catheter size (F)*	*Length (cm)**	*Guidewire (cm)*
Single Lumen			
21	2	04/06/08	20
20	3	08/15	20
19	4	10/20	30
18	5	15/20	30
16	7	15/20	30
Double Lumen			
19	4 (20G /22G)	06/10/15/20	50
18	5 (18G/20G)	06/15/20	50
16	7 (16G/18G)	15/20/30	50
Triple Lumen			
18	5 (18G/20G/20G)	06/10/15/20	50
16	7 (16G/18G/18G)	15/20/30	50

*Options of different lengths are available

Technique

Place the patient supine in Trendelenburg position (i.e. 15°–30° angle head down position) to make the IJV more prominent and prevent against dangerous air embolism which may occur during the procedure. Pillows that cause flexion of the neck should be removed, place a rolled towel under the shoulders for slight extension of neck and put arms by the side. Rotate the head to the opposite side but not greater than 45° as excess rotation increases the overlap of the internal jugular vein with the carotid artery and is associated with a higher risk of carotid puncture. Liver compression maneuver and simulated Valsalva maneuver (positive inspiratory pressure of 25 mm Hg for 10 seconds by inflating the reservoir bag) will increase the diameter of the internal jugular vein. Strict asepsis is to be maintained during the whole procedure.

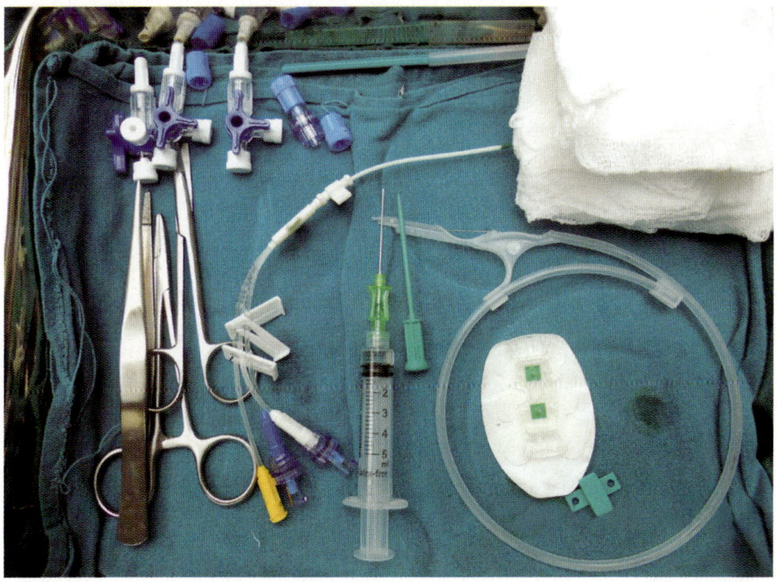

Fig. 2.4: Central venous catheter kit

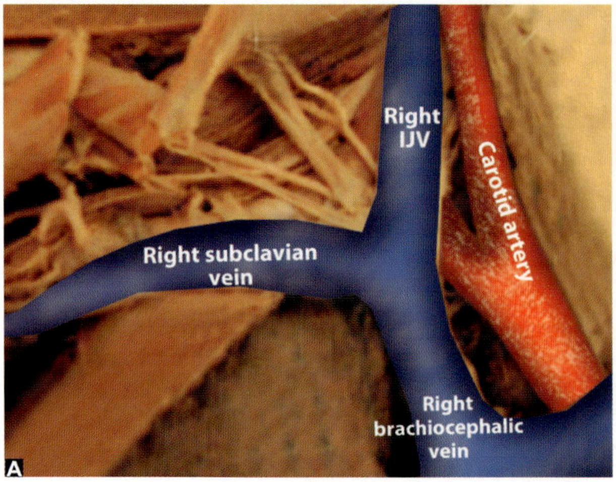

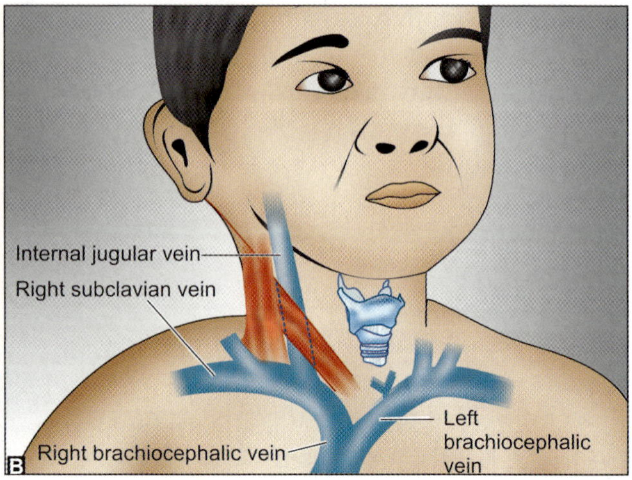

Figs 2.5A and B: (A) IJV anatomy; (B) Surface anatomy of IJV

Approaches

The IJV lies behind the internal carotid artery (ICA) in the upper part of the neck, lateral to the ICA in the middle third of the neck and anterolateral to the ICA in the lower neck joining the ipsilateral subclavian vein **(Figs 2.5A and B)**. The different approaches are **(Fig. 2.6)**:

- *Central approach* **(Fig. 2.7)**: Define the triangle formed by the two heads of the sternocleidomastoid muscle. Puncture at the apex at an angle of 30 to 45°, lateral to the carotid impulse and direct it towards ipsilateral nipple.
- *Central inferior approach (Low approach)* **(Fig. 2.8)**: The needle is inserted at the center point of the triangle mentioned above at 30° angle to the skin in a caudad direction just lateral to the carotid impulse.
- *Anterior approach* **(Fig. 2.9)**: The pulsation of the carotid artery should be felt exactly at the mid-point between the mastoid process and sternal notch. The needle is inserted at 45° angle to the skin just lateral to the carotid impulse in direction of the ipsilateral nipple.

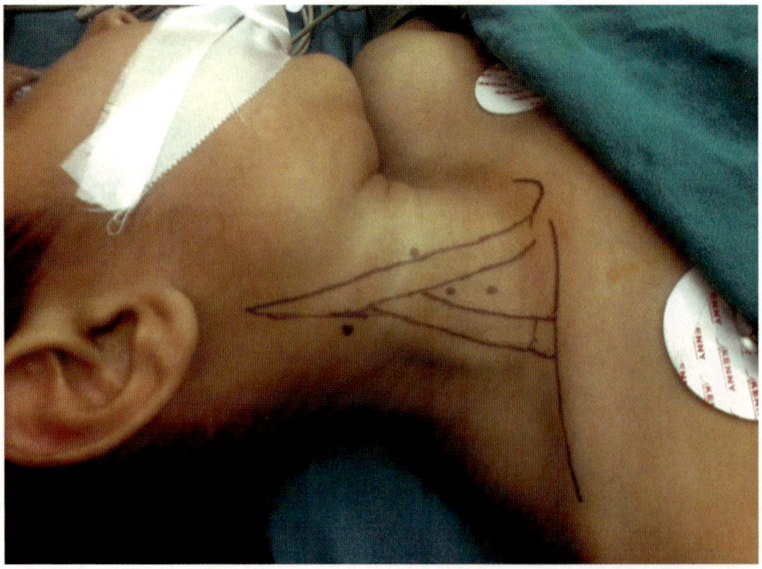

Fig. 2.6: Different approaches of IJV cannulation

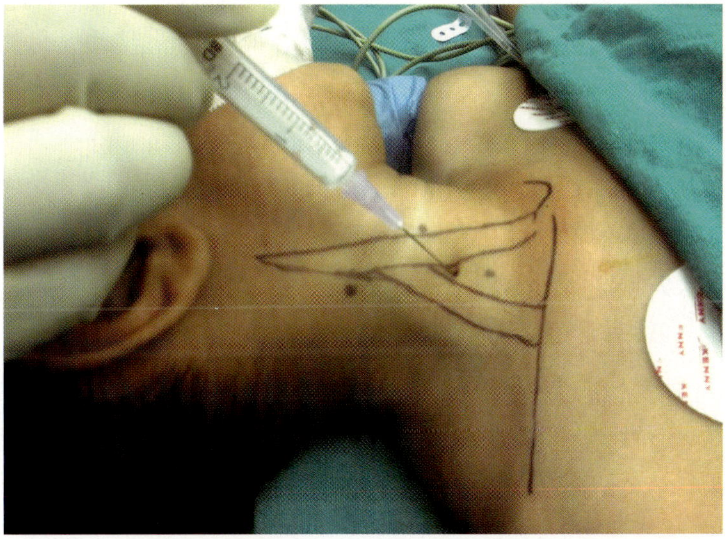

Fig. 2.7: Central approach

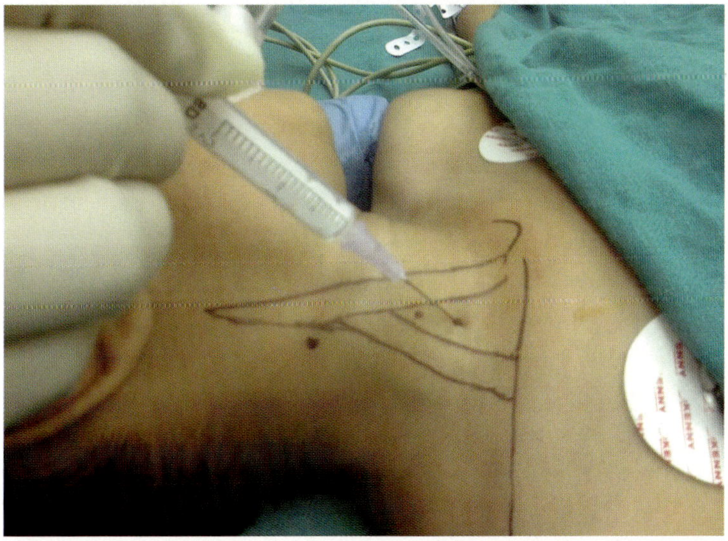

Fig. 2.8: Central inferior approach

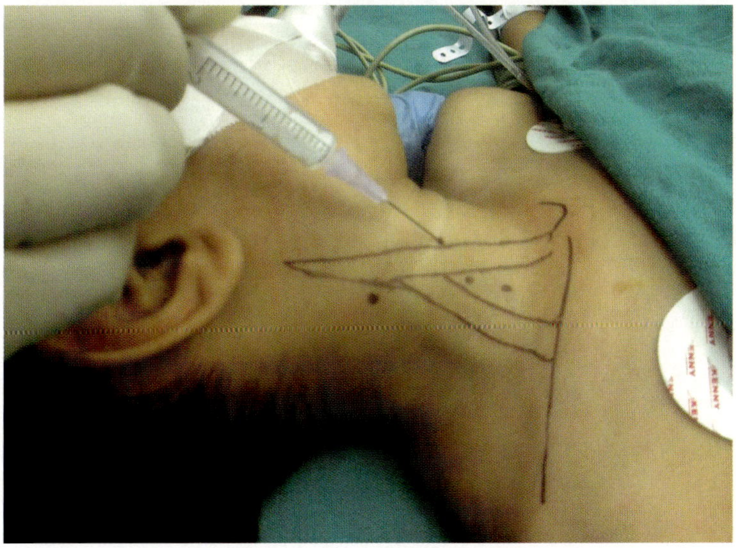

Fig. 2.9: Anterior approach

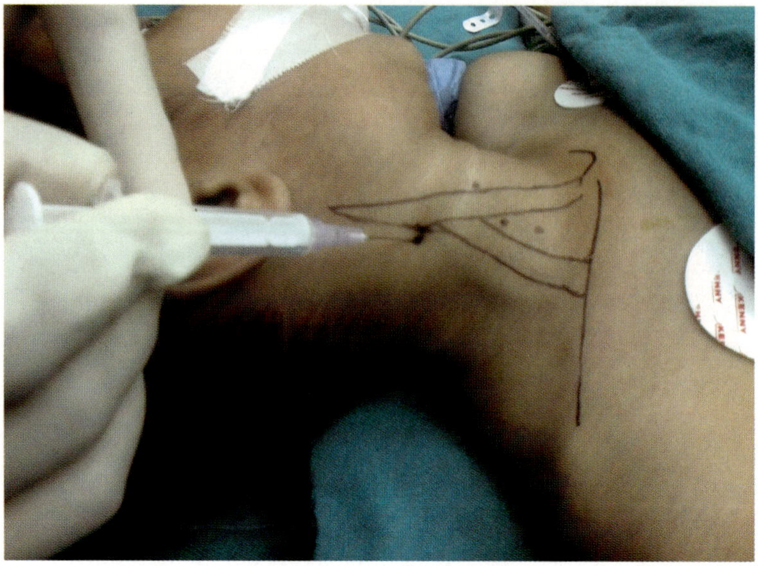

Fig. 2.10: Posterior approach

- *Posterior approach (High approach)* **(Fig. 2.10)**: With the upper border of the thyroid cartilage as the landmark, puncture just lateral to the carotid impulse where the external jugular vein crosses the lateral border of the sternocleidomastoid muscle. The needle points towards the sternal notch. The advantage of this approach is availability of a longer length of vein and avoidance of the danger of pneumothorax.

A 22G needle is used to locate the IJV, then a larger needle attached to a syringe filled with heparinized saline is inserted in the same location and advanced with continuous aspiration in the same direction as the finder needle. The finder needle may not be required when the access needle is smaller than 20G.

Once the needle is in the lumen of the vein (after two tissue-pops are felt; one at the prevertebral fascia and the other at the vein wall), dark venous blood is aspirated. Gently detach the syringe after fixing the needle with your hand against the patient. The guidewire should be ready and within easy reach, so that the needle does not move out of vein. The guidewire should pass through the needle without much resistance. If some resistance is felt, try to rotate the needle a bit, in case it abuts against the vein wall. Otherwise remove the guidewire and needle together and reattempt the puncture. The Seldinger technique (threading of catheter over guidewire) is used for insertion of the catheter **(Fig. 2.11)**.

Advantage

Compressibility of the IJV is possible in the event of an arterial puncture.

Complications

- Arterial puncture or cannulation
- Pneumothorax
- Hemothorax
- Nerve injuries
- Arrhythmia
- Air embolization
- Infection

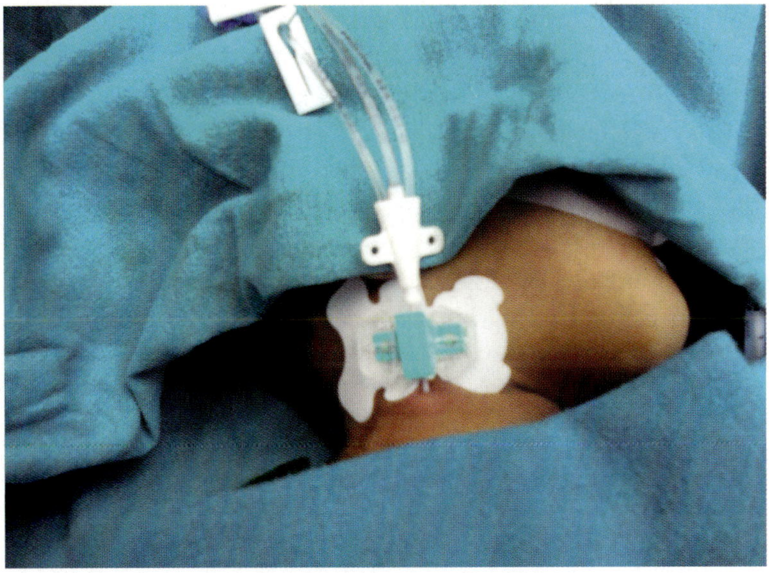

Fig. 2.11: IJV cannula *in situ*

- Venous thrombosis
- Embolization of guidewire or catheter
- Less comfortable, especially in tracheostomized children.

SUBCLAVIAN VEIN CANNULATION

The subclavian vein (SCV) is located immediately behind the medial third of the clavicle **(Figs 2.12A and B)**. It is less frequently used in neonates as technically, it is more difficult. In case of accidental arterial puncture, difficulty in obtaining hemostasis in neonates may prove fatal.

Technique

This option is considered only if all other sites have been exhausted. The right subclavian is the first choice as the dome of the lung is more cephalad on the left side and also the thoracic duct is placed on the left side. A small rolled gauze is placed vertically between the shoulders so that they droop posteriorly. The patient is placed supine in the Trendelenburg position with arms by the side, thus optimizing the length of the subclavian vein overlapped by the clavicle. Turn the

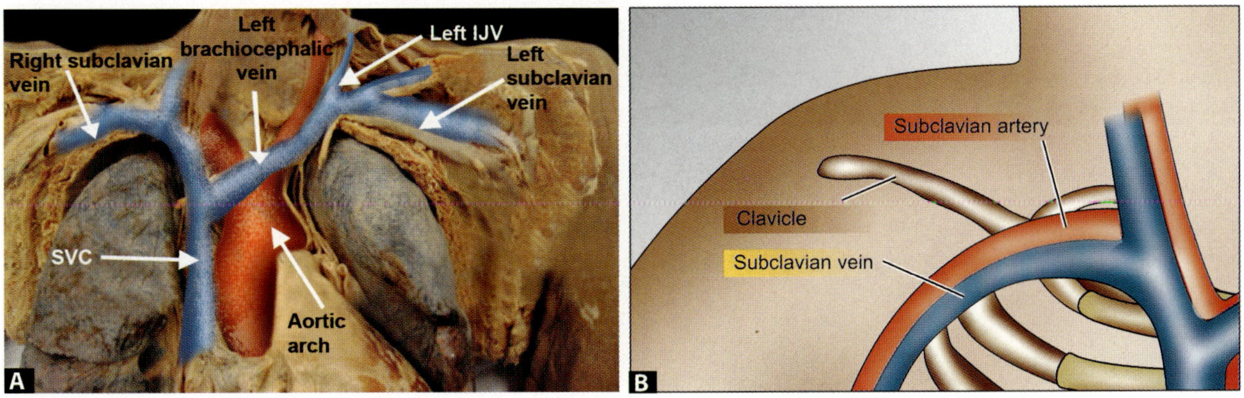

Figs 2.12A and B: Subclavian vein anatomy

head to the ipsilateral side to compress the internal jugular vein of the same side and prevent the guidewire from entering the IJV, especially in infants.

Strict asepsis is a must. Puncture with an introducer needle at the junction of the medial and middle one-third of the clavicle in the depression between the deltoid and pectoralis major. Contact the clavicle with the needle and walk it underneath the bone with constant aspiration until venous blood is aspirated. Advance the needle only during expiration. The needle should be parallel to the chest wall and directed posteriorly, medially and slightly cephalad towards sternal notch. Use a dilator, but do not advance too far, to prevent puncture of the vein wall. The CV catheter is introduced using the Seldinger technique.

While slowly advancing the guidewire through the needle look for premature atrial contractions (PACs) which indicate that it is in the right atrium. If no PACs are seen even after insertion of a sufficient length of guidewire, its misplacement into ipsilateral IJV is a likely possibility. Then withdraw the guidewire and rotate by 90° clockwise with J-tip downward and advance the guidewire until PACs are seen. Then it should be withdrawn a little so that it lies outside the right atrium. The catheter is then secured in place and a sterile transparent dressing applied. Subcutaneous tunnelling of the subclavian line can be done when 8 cm or longer line is used for better placement and secure fixation.

Caution

- Pleural entry can be detected when air is aspirated through the needle
- Confirm position of catheter radiologically – ideal position of tip of catheter is at junction of SVC and right atrium **(Figs 2.13A and B)**
- Continuous pulse oximetry monitoring should be done
- Watch for sudden desaturation and auscultate for bilateral equal breath sounds
- Keep chest-tube tray ready.

Advantages

- Constant position of SCV in reference to surface landmarks at all ages
- More comfortable for the patient
- Lower incidence of catheter colonization and bacteremia.

Disadvantages

- Occasional inability to expand space between first rib and clavicle
- 5-20% incidence of malposition

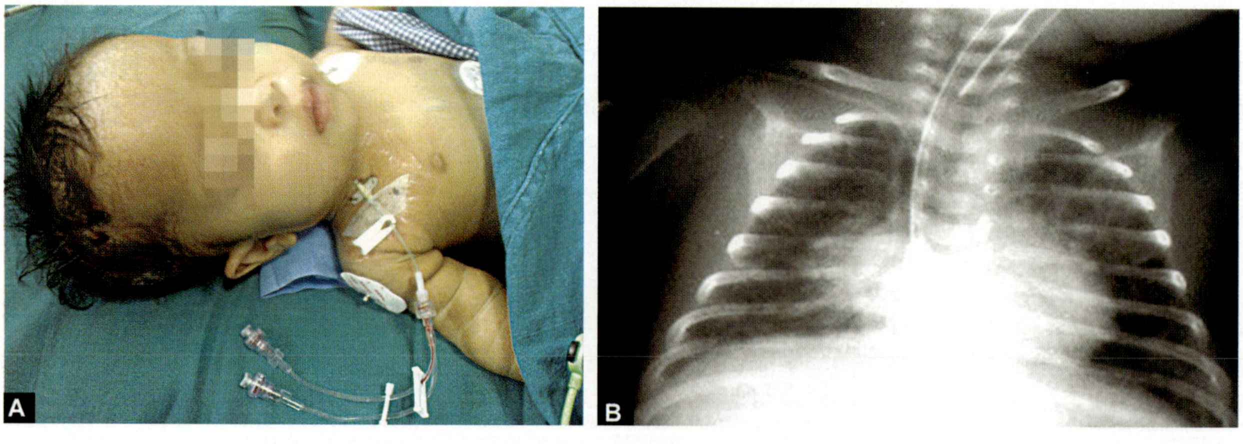

Figs 2.13A and B: (A) SCV catheter *in situ;* (B) Radiological confirmation

- No arterial pulsations for landmark
- The smaller the baby, the more the chance of complication.

Complications

- Pneumothorax
- Arterial puncture
- Infection
- Thrombosis
- Thoracic duct injury
- Brachial plexus damage
- Migration into the IJV
- Hemothorax.

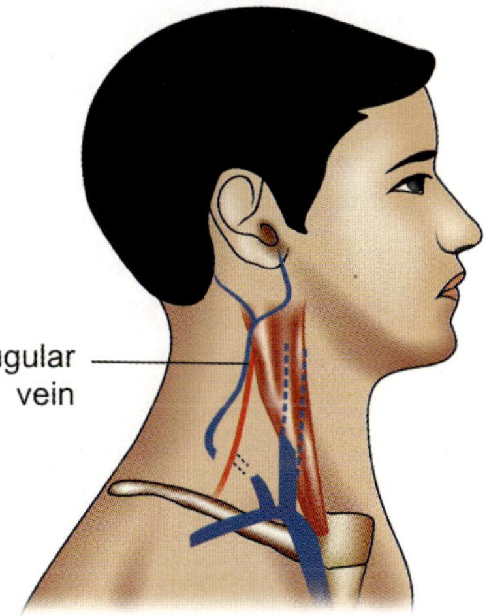

Fig. 2.14: External jugular vein anatomy

EXTERNAL JUGULAR VEIN CANNULATION

The external jugular vein (EJV) runs through the neck from the angle of the mandible to join the subclavian vein at an acute angle behind the middle of the clavicle, crossing the sternocleidomastoid muscle en route **(Fig. 2.14)**. It is a superficial structure, variable in size and has valves.

Indication

Where IJV/SCV cannot be successfully cannulated.

Technique

External jugular vein (EJV) cannulation should be done preferably on the right side under strict asepsis. A rolled towel under the shoulder causes a slight extension of the neck and rotation of the head 45–90° away from the side of cannulation provides optimal position. A 30° Trendelenburg position distends the vein and an assistant should directly compress the vein gently just over the clavicle to make it prominent for easy cannulation **(Figs 2.15A and B)**.

Insert the needle with an attached heparinized saline filled syringe at 10–20° angle with traction of the overlying skin where the vein is most easily seen. Caution should be exercised as such a position may cause potential compromise of the airway in very small babies. The higher the point of cannulation, the lower the risk of pneumothorax. A short peripheral cannula may be used for access, the needle is removed and the cannula is used for the Seldinger technique for a CVC placement. Sometimes passing a guidewire may be difficult because of the presence of a valve which is usually present at the point where the EJV penetrates the fascia to empty into the subclavian vein. In this situation, manipulation of the shoulder can facilitate the passage of the guidewire. A J-point guidewire is preferable to a straight guidewire. The proper position of the guidewire in the right atrium is confirmed by the appearance of PACs as in SCV cannulation. The catheter should preferably be sutured in place.

Advantages

- Superficial location
- Easy access
- Low risk of arterial puncture.

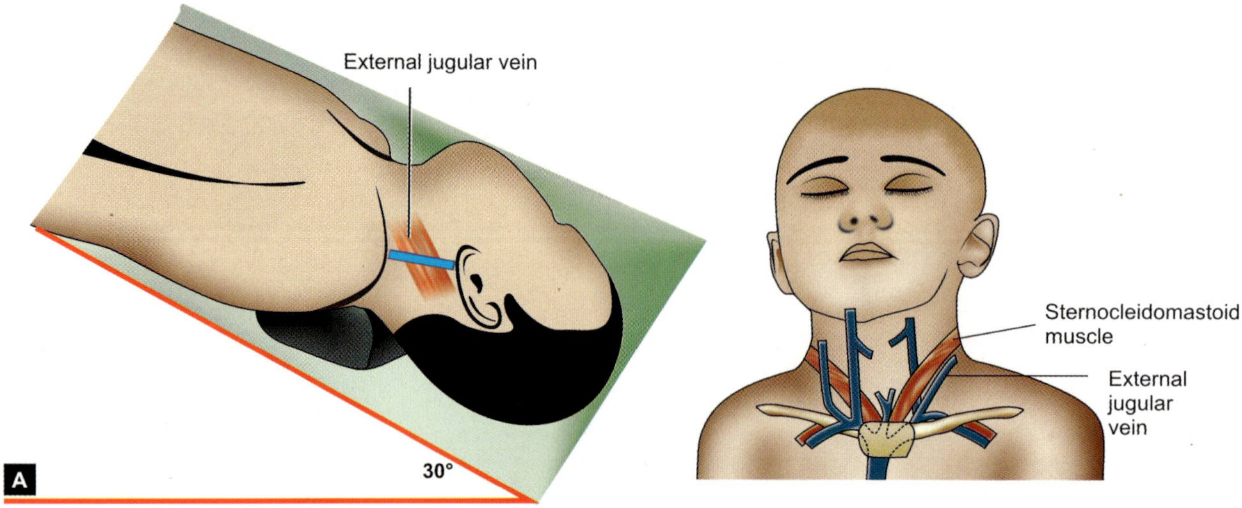

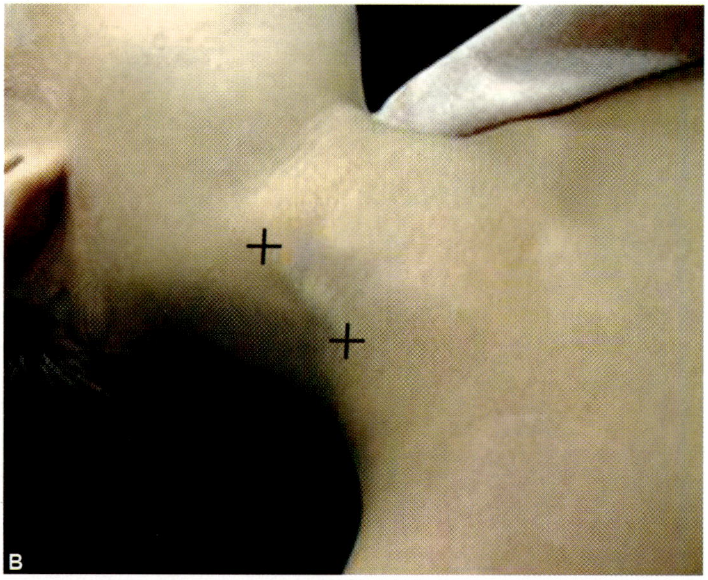

Figs 2.15A and B: (A) Optimal position for EJV cannulation; (B) Surface landmark

Disadvantages

- The younger the child, the less likely that the EJV catheter would enter the RA
- Low success rate.

FEMORAL VEIN CANNULATION

The femoral vein lies medial to the femoral artery in the femoral triangle below the inguinal ligament. Superficial and deep fascial layers separate the femoral vein from the skin **(Figs 2.16A and B)**.

Indications

- Inability to cannulate peripheral veins
- Infusion of irritant drugs or potent vasoconstrictors

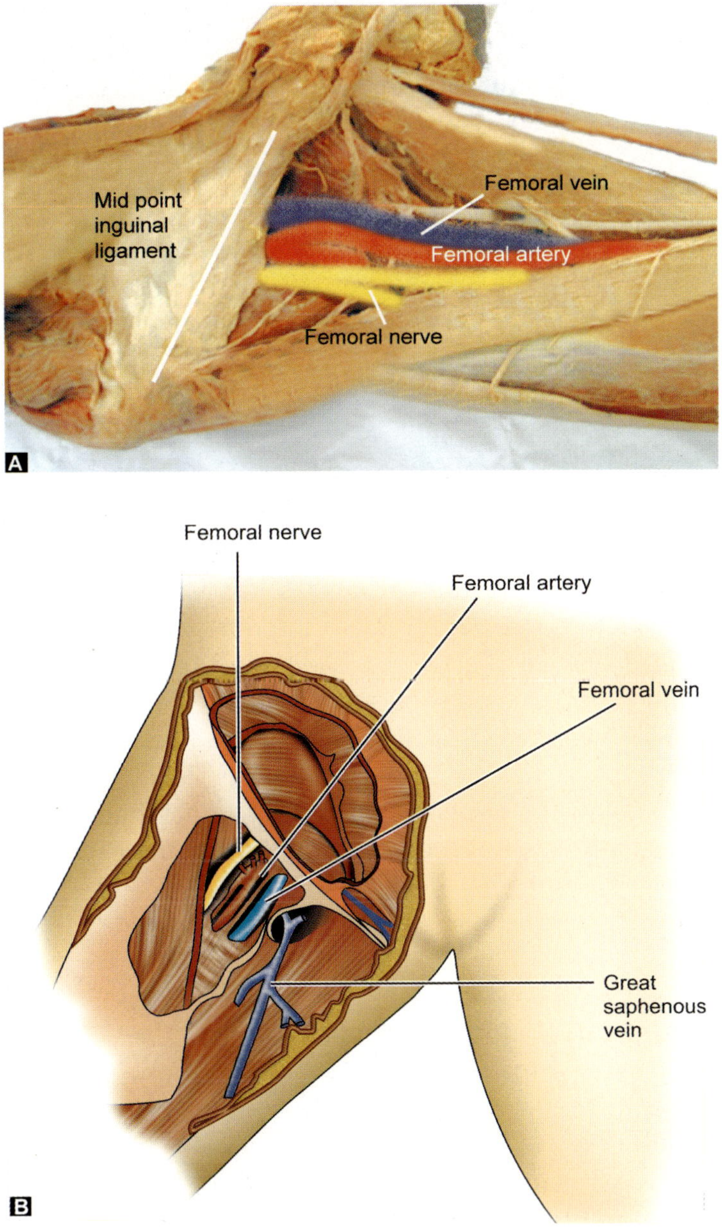

Figs 2.16A and B: Femoral vein anatomy

- Frequent sampling when arterial line is not accessible
- TPN or large volume of fluid administration.

Contraindications

- Hematoma, thrombus or abscess at site of puncture
- Limb deformity where distorted vascular anatomy is a possibility
- Vascular insufficiency of extremity
- Deranged coagulation profile.

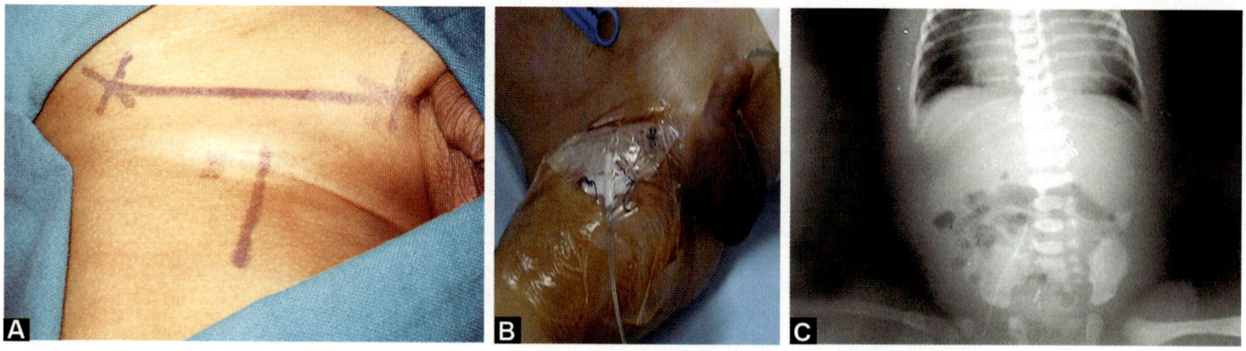

Figs 2.17A to C: (A) Surface landmark; (B) Femoral vein catheter *in situ*; (C) Radiological confirmation

Technique

Strict asepsis is a essential. The child is placed supine with a rolled towel under hip and leg is externally rotated. The right femoral vein is preferred as it is easier to approach from the right side for a right-handed operator and the catheter is less likely to migrate into the posterior lumbar venous plexus. Puncture the vein 1-2 cm inferior to the inguinal ligament, 0.5-1 cm medial to the femoral artery while the needle is directed towards the umbilicus at a 30-45° angle. Ultrasound guidance improves the success rate. The Seldinger technique is used with insertion of a guidewire, followed by the definitive catheter. Pass the catheter all the way to the hub. Sterile transparent dressing should be applied **(Figs 2.17A to C)**.

Femoral vein puncture below the inguinal ligament prevents the formation of retroperitoneal hematoma. Catheter placement is confirmed by X-ray. Ideally the catheter should be above the diaphragm.

Advantages

- Relatively easy with fewer complications
- Femoral arterial pulse provides good landmark
- Easily compressible in case of inadvertent arterial puncture
- Preferred in patients with single ventricle
- Does not interfere with CPR
- Left side is preferred in patients expected to undergo multiple interventions
- Can be performed with mild sedation and local analgesia.

Disadvantages

- Difficult to maintain sterility
- Higher rate of catheter colonization and clinical sepsis
- Femoral nerve injury
- Air embolism
- Risk of femoral artery puncture and formation of hematoma
- Limb edema
- Bladder perforation
- Thrombosis of femoral vein
- Peritoneal perforation
- Septic arthritis
- Vein rupture leading to abdominal distention and peritonitis

Table 2.2: Available sizes of PICC

Introducer size	*Catheter size*	*Length (cm)*	*Flow rate gravity (cc/hr)*
24 G	1F/28 G	20	30
22 G	1.9F/26 G	30	35
20 G	2.8F/22 G	50	310
19 G	3F/20 G	65	130
17 G	4F/18 G	65	270
15 G	5 F/16 G	65	560
	5 F/(16 G-16 G) (double)	65	150
	5 F/(18 G-19 G-19 G) (Triple)	40/45/50/55	

- Unreliable drug delivery in low flow states
- Poor patient mobility
- Unreliable CVP monitoring.

PERIPHERALLY INSERTED CENTRAL CATHETER (PICC) PLACEMENT

Advanced neonatal care has led to the improved survival of preterm and low birth weight babies. They have a longer stay in nursery and a need for long-term vascular access. PICC line insertion is one of the safest and most popular techniques for this purpose.

A PICC line is inserted in a large peripheral vein and then advanced through increasingly larger veins, towards the heart until the tip reaches in the distal superior vena cava or cava-atrial junction **(Table 2.2)**.

Indications

- Difficult peripheral venous access
- Prolonged intravenous fluid/antibiotic/chemotherapy
- TPN, high concentration dextrose infusion
- Preterm, extremely low birth weight (ELBW) babies
- Hemodynamic monitoring.

Contraindications

- Anatomical irregularity in extremities
- Broken skin or infection at site of insertion.

Technique

This vascular access is for short-to-intermediate term use. The highest success rate is with the basilic vein though cephalic vein, saphenous vein, popliteal vein, axillary vein can also be used. The key to success is to attempt PICC placement before large, visible peripheral veins are injured. Strict asepsis must be maintained throughout the procedure even if it is done at the bedside.

Insertable portion of a PICC varies from 20 to 60 cm in length (i.e. adequate to reach the desired tip position in most patients). Guidewire option is available to stiffen the PICC for

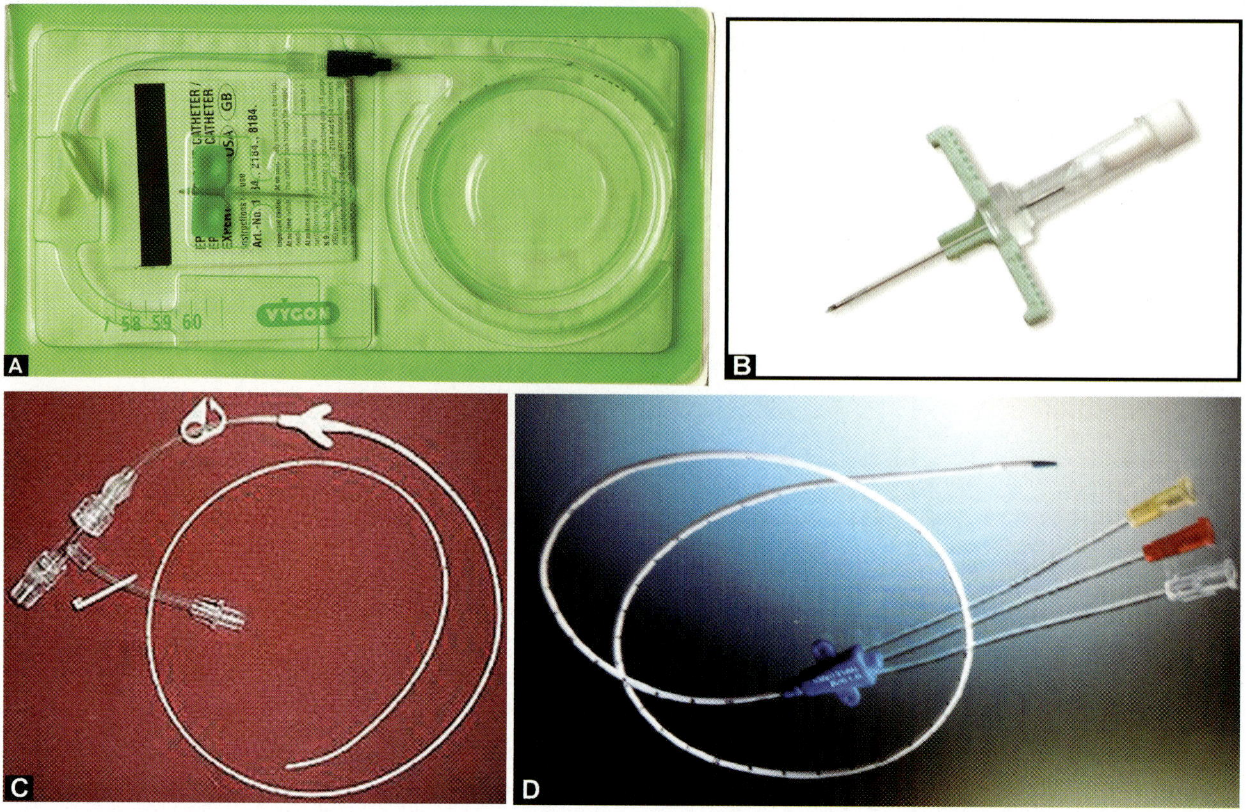

Figs 2.18A to D: (A) PICC; (B) PICC introducer; (C) PICC with extended hub; (D) Triple lumen PICC

easy insertion through the veins. The introducers or sheaths are available separately or "peel-away" type. The soft, strong silicone shaft material provides tissue-friendly long-term care. They are also available in thermosensitive polyurethane material which is easier to insert, yet softens after placement **(Figs 2.18A to D)**.

Accurate catheter positioning needs measurement from site of insertion to xiphisternum. The catheter is passed with an iris forceps through the introducer till the calculated distance. It should pass easily without resistance and with continuous aspiration of blood. Only 5 ml or 10 ml syringe should be used as increased pressure at the tip with 1 or 2 ml syringe can rupture the lines. While inserting the catheter the points of resistance are the main joints (shoulder joint, knee joint, hip joint). To overcome this, abduct and straighten the joint, push heparinized solution while slowly advancing the catheter. If the catheter does not cross the major joints, then it is not a central line and such a line is more likely to get thrombosed. Ultrasound, chest radiography and fluoroscopy aid in their insertion and confirm placement (due to barium sulfate loaded catheter body). The tip should never be in the heart, because of the risk of perforation and cardiac tamponade.

The proximal portion has a wing with holes for suturing to prevent accidental removal. It may also have an extended hub option which minimizes skin irritation and makes it convenient for clinical access. A transparent dressing should be applied as the insertion site should be visible **(Figs 2.19A and B)**. The IV fluid should always be connected otherwise it gets blocked because of small lumen. At the time of its removal, the length should be measured up to the hub and recorded in the patient's chart which should tally with the documentation done at insertion.

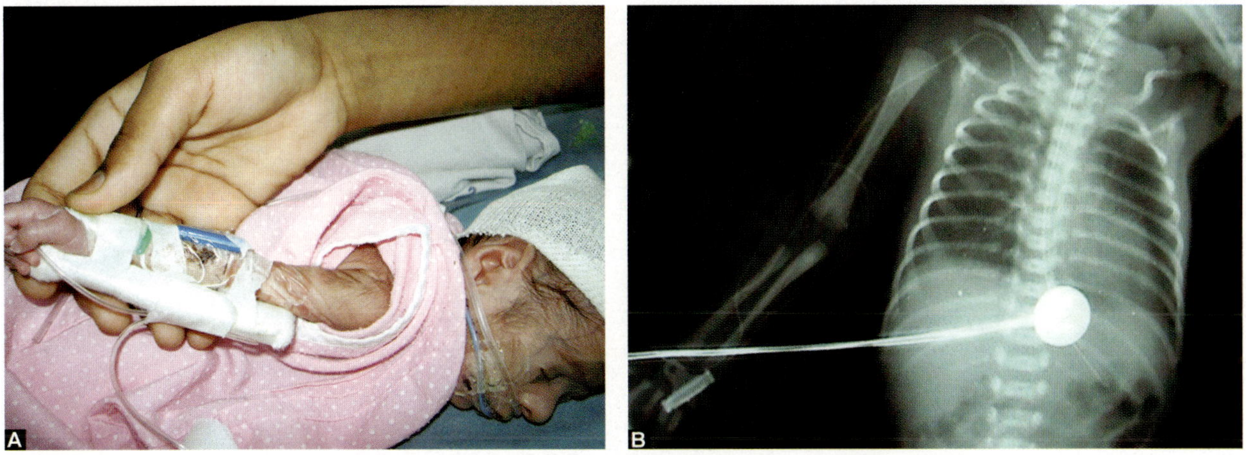

Figs 2.19A and B: (A) PICC *in situ;* (B) PICC in right cephalic vein

Merits

- Easy to insert, a bed-side procedure
- Reliable venous access
- Multiple insertion site choices
- Used for prolonged period ($\leq$ 30 days)
- Relatively inexpensive
- Lower rate of infection
- No risk of pneumothorax.

Demeritis

- Potential for catheter occlusion
- Leaking lines due to punctured lumen
- Catheter embolization following shearing
- Sepsis, phlebitis, thrombosis, air embolism
- Difficult to position in central vein
- Atrial perforation, cardiac tamponade.

Routine Care of PICC Line

- Prophylactic heparin reduces chances of occlusion, i.e. heparin @ 1 unit/hr
- Routine dressing change is not recommended due to risk of contamination and accidental dislodgement. It should be changed only if indicated (i.e. kinked, evidence of inflammation or bleeding at insertion site)
- Minimize the numbers of connections as much as possible
- Catheter tips are sent for microbiological examination, when removed because of sepsis.

Indications for Removal of Catheter

- Local infection at insertion site
- Septicemia
- Evidence of septic emboli or endocarditis
- Bacteremia persisting beyond 48-72 hr despite appropriate antibiotic therapy.

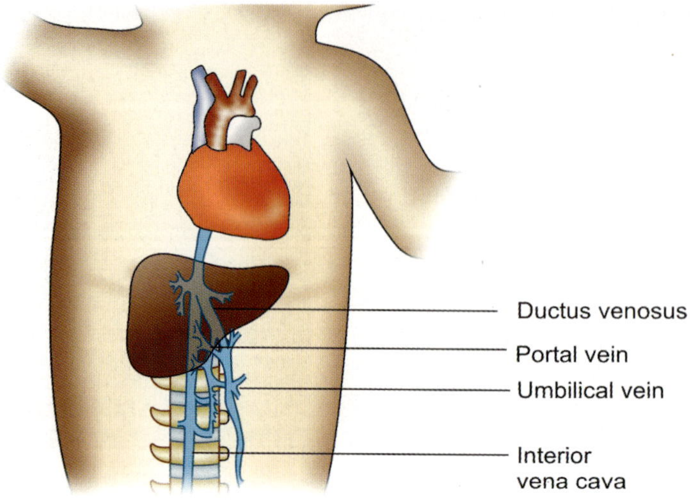

Fig. 2.20: Course of the umbilical vein

UMBILICAL VENOUS CATHETERIZATION (UVC)

It is a rapid and reliable access to the vascular system of critically ill neonates. UV closure usually occurs after closure of umbilical artery (UA) and remains patent for approximately 1 week after birth. UV is 2-3 cm long, 4-5 mm in diameter and then joins the left portal vein and ductus venosus **(Fig. 2.20)**.

Indications

- Resuscitation—administration of drugs like adrenaline and vasoactive drugs
- Infusion of hypertonic solutions (greater than 10% concentration of glucose)
- Initial delivery of parenteral nutrition until percutaneous central venous access is established
- Delivery of blood and blood products – however, platelets preferably should not be administered via this route
- Measurement of central venous pressure
- Exchange transfusion
- Frequent blood sampling in an unstable patient.

Technique

Place newborn supine under radiant warmer and initiate pulse oximetry, temperature and cardiorespiratory monitoring. Document bruising of lower extremities prior to placement of UVC. For active infants, restrain the legs and arms. Clean the stump and adjoining abdomen with iodine solution and sterile draping is done. Place a cord tie loosely around the base of the cord to secure hemostasis and cut the cord 1-1.5 cm above the skin line. The tie should not be too tight to prevent the passage of catheter Take care that the cut surface is not ragged **(Figs 2.21A to C)**. Hold the stump upright. The umbilical vein is single, large, thin walled and usually at 12 o'clock position; whereas the umbilical arteries are two, small, thick walled and tightly constricted. The position of vessels may differ depending on where the cord is cut as the vessels circle around the cord.

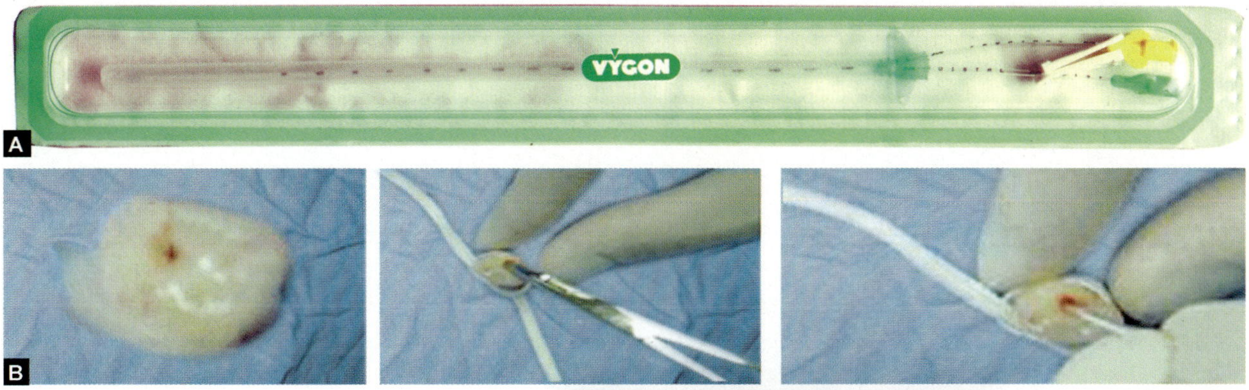

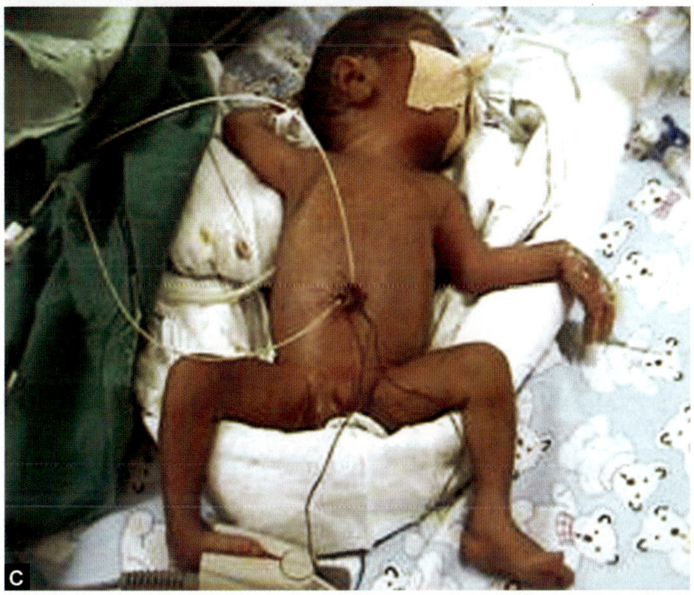

Figs 2.21A to C: (A) Umbilical vein cannula; (B) Umbilical vein cannulation; (C) UVC *in situ*

Identify the vein and remove any visible clot. Insert the catheter tip and advance it towards the pelvis. Use umbilical catheter of following sizes:

- Preterm < 1500 gm – 3.5F,
  >1500 gm – 5F,
- Term – 6F.

A feeding tube option should be the last resort. A multiport catheter with provision for measurement of venous oxygen saturation is also available which should be used for critically ill neonates requiring simultaneous multiple infusion. Connect the catheter to a pressure transducer before connecting to the vein. Never open the catheter to the atmosphere, insert while continuously measuring the pressure.

On crossing the ductus venosus and reaching the IVC, there is a sudden drop in pressure and the waveform will resemble an atrial pressure tracing. Once in the thorax, measure the pO_2. If pO_2 >50 mm Hg it is in the left atrium or pulmonary vein. Ventricular waveform indicates its presence in left ventricle. Withdraw the catheter till waveform with dominant 'a' wave appears (right atrium) and blood color changes to less pink and shows negative deflections with respiration. It is better to position the catheter too high and withdraw as necessary according to location on X-ray as the line can not be advanced once the sterile technique is broken. Do not nurse infant prone or place in a nappy for 4 hours after removal of UVC.

Table 2.3: Sizes of umbilical catheter

Size (F)	*Length (cm)*	*ID (mm)*	*OD (mm)*	*Flow rate ml/min*	*Priming volume (ml)*
Single lumen					
2.5	30	0.5	0.8	2.35	0.21
3.5	40	0.8	1.2	11.1	0.34
4	40	0.8	1.5	11.3	0.36
5	40	1.0	1.7	23	0.46
8	40	1.5	2.5	79	0.84
Double lumen					
4 (20G/20G)	20		1.4	15	0.26
4 (20G/20G)	40		1.4	6	0.28
5 (19G/19G)	40		1.7	9	0.3

Length of insertion (cm) = 1.5 x BW(kg) + 5.6 cm

This formula may overestimate the required length but gives a good guide **(Table 2.3)**.

Location of Catheter Tip

Possible locations for UVC tip are umbilical vein, portal vein, portal sinus, RA, LA, LV, pulmonary vein and SVC **(Figs 2.22A to C)**.

a. Preferred positions:
   - Low—beyond ductus venosus in IVC, i.e. just above aortic bifurcation between L_3 and L_4 vertebrae. Insert 4–6 cm for resuscitation or exchange transfusion
   - High—tip should be 0.5-1.5 cm above the diaphragm and below the right atrium in the vena cava for indwelling use, i.e. between T_6 and T_9 vertebrae. This placement is associated with fewer ischemic and thrombotic complications. There occurs negative pressure deflections during spontaneous respiration and during deep inspiration or sigh, the pressure goes well below atmospheric pressure (about -10 mm Hg). It is not desirable to place it in the portal venous systems as pressures are higher and variable.

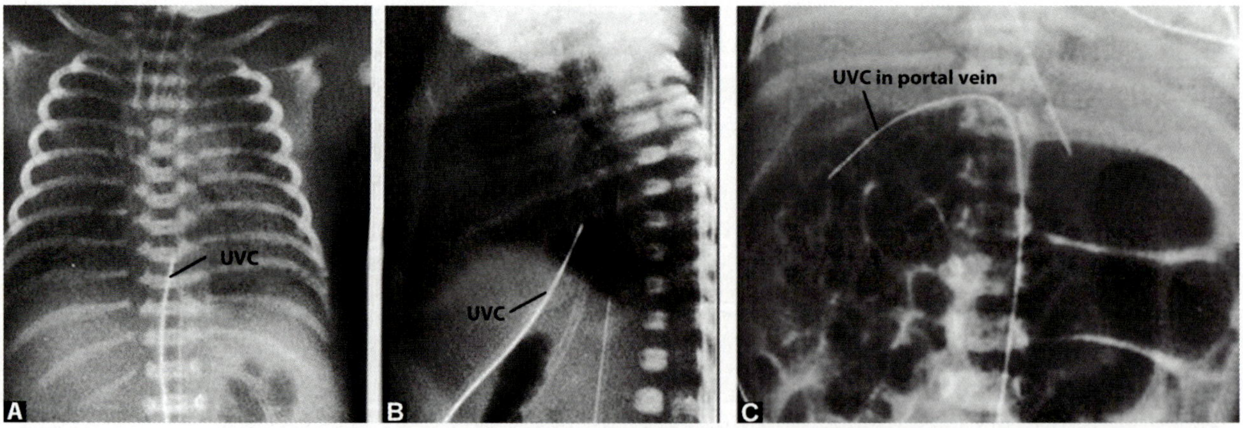

Figs 2.22A to C: (A and B) Radiological confirmation; (C) UVC in portal vein

In this situation, the mean pressure is higher than CVP and the pressure goes slightly positive during inspiration and never goes below atmospheric pressure or zero. The problems associated with portal placement are:
- Infusion of hypertonic solutions (10% dextrose or $NaHCO_3$) may produce thrombosis of portal vessels or hepatic necrosis
- Exchange transfusion into portal vessels may cause obstruction of portal venous flow causing necrotizing enterocolitis.

b. The tip should not be allowed to crossover to left side because of risk of systemic embolism
c. Confirm the location by pressure and pO_2 measurements and chest radiograph (never by the length of catheter insertion)
d. Fluids should not be administered until radiological confirmation is obtained.

Complications of UVC

- Infection
- Blood loss due to accidental disconnection
- Potentially catastrophic air embolism if bubbles infused or catheter system is open to atmosphere
- Portal venous thrombosis
- Necrotizing enterocolitis
- Catheter malposition.

Contraindications

- Omphalitis
- Omphalocele
- Necrotizing enterocolitis
- Peritonitis
- Evidence of vascular compromise in lower limbs.

Ascertainment of Correct Position of Central Venous Catheters (CVCs)

- *Post-procedural chest radiograph* is the gold standard to assess complications and catheter positions. An AP radiograph of chest and upper abdomen is taken to identify the tip of the catheter.
- *TEE* detects position of guidewires and catheter tips with 100% success rate whereas it is 86% with surface landmarks. CVC is positioned 1-2 cm above crista terminalis. Proximal SVC is difficult to image with TEE, so this method is most accurate in placing CVC in distal SVC.
- Intravascular ECG is used as a guide while advancing the catheter and guidewire. Entry into RA is marked by appearance of P-atriale. Thereafter the catheter is pulled out by 1-2 cm into SVC. Success rate is 80-90% but it requires specialized equipment.

PERIPHERAL VENOUS CUTDOWN

The surgical venous cutdown still has a limited role in emergency situation when other peripheral and IO attempts fail. Saphenous vein anterior to the medial malleolus of tibia is the most popular choice for this access. Antecubital and femoral vessels can also be of use. The distal end of the vein is typically ligated, therefore, the vein is precluded from use as future vascular access. A venotomy is made carefully with a number 11 blade to avoid complete transsection of vein.

Arterial Cannulation

INDICATIONS

- Evaluation of respiratory and acid-base status
- Patients requiring assisted ventilation
- Shock, intoxication, metabolic derangement
- Routine laboratory analysis if venous sampling not possible
- To guide fluid and inotrope administration
- Invasive continuous blood pressure monitoring
- Exchange transfusion.

SITES

- *Central artery*
  - *Umbilical artery*
- *Peripheral artery*
  - *Commonly used*
    Radial artery
    Posterior tibial artery
  - *Occasionally used*
    Dorsalis pedis artery
    Ulnar artery
  - *Rarely used*
    Axillary artery
- Avoid femoral and brachial arteries (due to poor collaterals) and temporal artery because of possible CNS damage due to retrograde embolism.

Peripheral arterial catheters are indicated when:

- UAC unsuccessful
- Infant too old for UAC
- Pre-ductal PaO_2 measurement (i.e. right radial artery) is indicated
- UAC already in place for several days or removed due to thrombus formation.

Advantages of peripheral arterial catheters:

- Can be used for several days
- Minor and infrequent complications.

EQUIPMENT

- 24G venipuncture cannula (for neonates)/scalp vein set /22G arterial cannula
- 1 ml syringe for blood gas sampling
- Pressure lines
- Heparinized saline (0.5–1.0 U/ml) in syringe-pump infused at 0.5 ml/hr in neonates for maintaining patency of artery
- Transilluminator.

TECHNIQUE

General

Under aseptic skin preparation the needle is positioned against direction of flow at an angle of 15°-25° with bevel downward for superficial artery and at an angle of 30°- 45° bevel upward for deep artery. Transillumination may assist location of the vessel. First penetrate skin, then puncture the artery. When bright red blood flows with pulsation, the catheter is advanced directly or via Seldinger technique. Then the catheter should be connected to the transducer.

Check for blood return, pulse waveform and adequacy of distal circulation. If the catheter cannot be advanced smoothly, it is not in the arterial lumen. In such a situation it should not be forced, but removed. If withdrawal is necessary, apply firm pressure at puncture site for 5 minutes and repeat skin preparation. In case of hematoma formation, it may not be possible to catheterize that artery.

Radial Artery Cannulation (Figs 2.23A to E)

Perform the Allen's test to assess adequate collateral circulation. Locate the radial and ulnar arteries at the proximal wrist crease. The radial artery lies lateral to the flexor carpi radialis tendon while the ulnar artery is medial to the flexor carpi ulnaris tendon. Elevate the infant's hand and occlude both radial and ulnar arteries at the wrist. Then massage the palm towards wrist to drain blood from the hand and blanch the palm. Release occlusion of the ulnar artery while still compressing the radial artery. If the color returns to the palm in less than 6 seconds, it indicates adequate arterial collaterals. The radial artery should not be cannulated if color return takes more than 10 seconds.

Extend the wrist to about 45° by keeping a rolled gauze under the wrist and securing the hand and fingers to a board. Then the arterial cannulation is done as described in the general technique above.

Dorsalis Pedis/Posterior Tibial Artery Cannulation (Figs 2.24A and B)

These sites are better avoided in patients expected to have peripheral vasoconstriction or vasomotor instability. For dorsalis pedis artery cannulation, plantarflex the foot and palpate for the artery between second and third metatarsal.

For posterior tibial artery cannulation, dorsiflex the foot and puncture at a steep angle between the medial malleolus and Achilles tendon. The Seldinger technique is used to insert the arterial cannula. Monitor the limb for vascular insufficiency.

Complications

- Vascular
  - Thrombus formation
  - Ischemia of limb **(Fig. 2.23E)**
  - Hemorrhage
- Perforation
  - Extravasation/hematoma/compartment syndrome
- Infection
- Embolism
- Accidental drug injection
- Damage to arterial wall—aneurysm formation

Caution: If pulse diminishes or there is a change of color of the limb and becomes cold, dusky with a poor capillary refill, remove arterial line immediately.

Umbilical Artery Catheterization (UAC)

It is an elective procedure. Unless immediate vascular access is required, insertion of the technically more difficult UAC prior to UVC insertion is preferable, as occasionally the cord stump needs

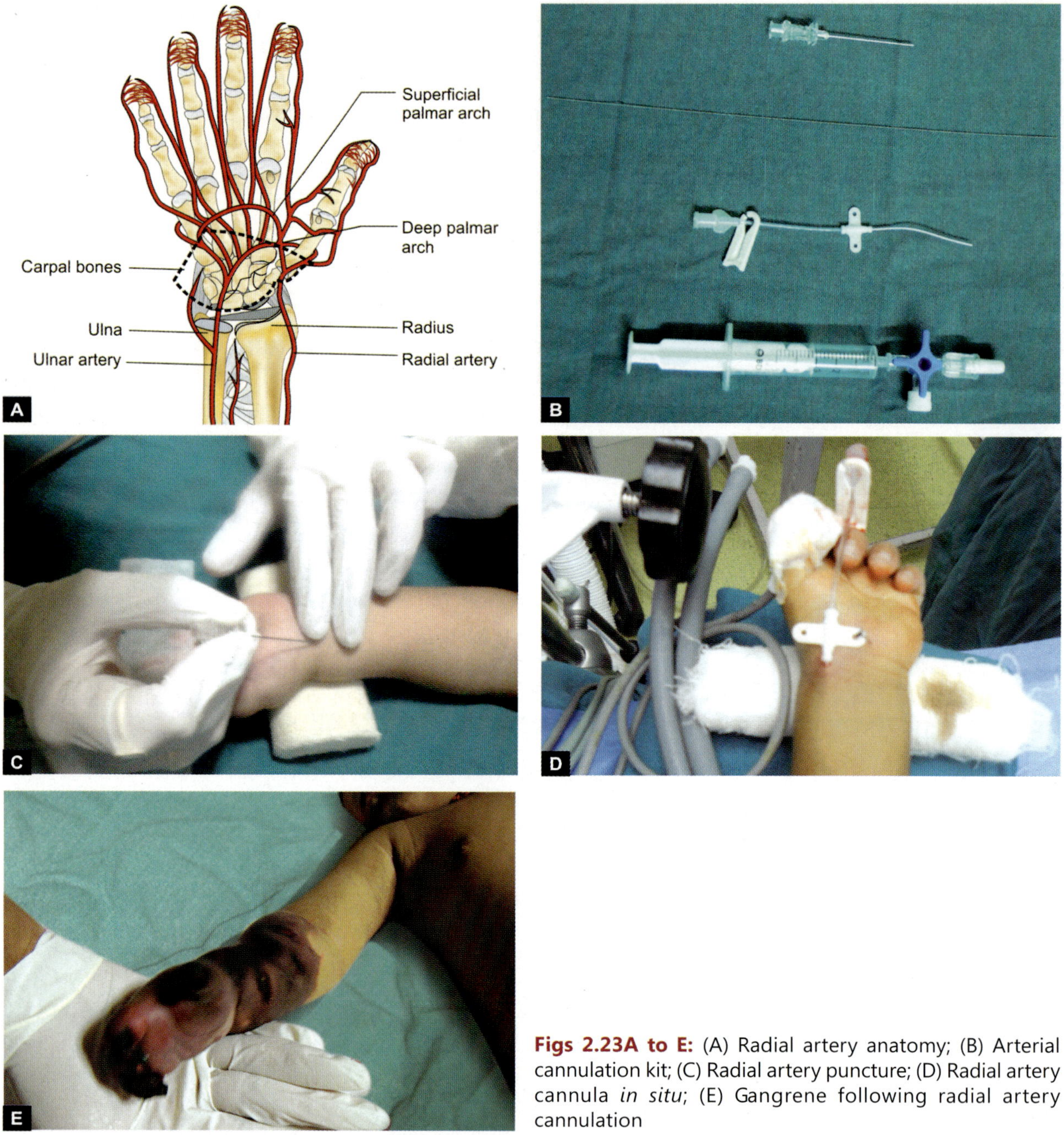

Figs 2.23A to E: (A) Radial artery anatomy; (B) Arterial cannulation kit; (C) Radial artery puncture; (D) Radial artery cannula *in situ*; (E) Gangrene following radial artery cannulation

to be recut to facilitate UAC insertion. The umbilical artery is readily accessible in the first few days of life. It gives accurate pressure monitoring as it is a large central artery. UAC is usually performed by neonatologists using 3.5 F catheter in children <1500 gm and 5.0 F catheter in children >1500 gm **(Figs 2.25A to D)**.

Technique: The umbilical arteries turn inferiorly towards the pelvis and join the internal iliac arteries. They begin to constrict within seconds after birth and functionally close within a few minutes. Insertion of a catheter can be attempted as long as the umbilical stump is attached, preferably within 3-4 days of life. In extremely low birth weight (ELBW) babies, UAC is better tolerated than a peripheral arterial line.

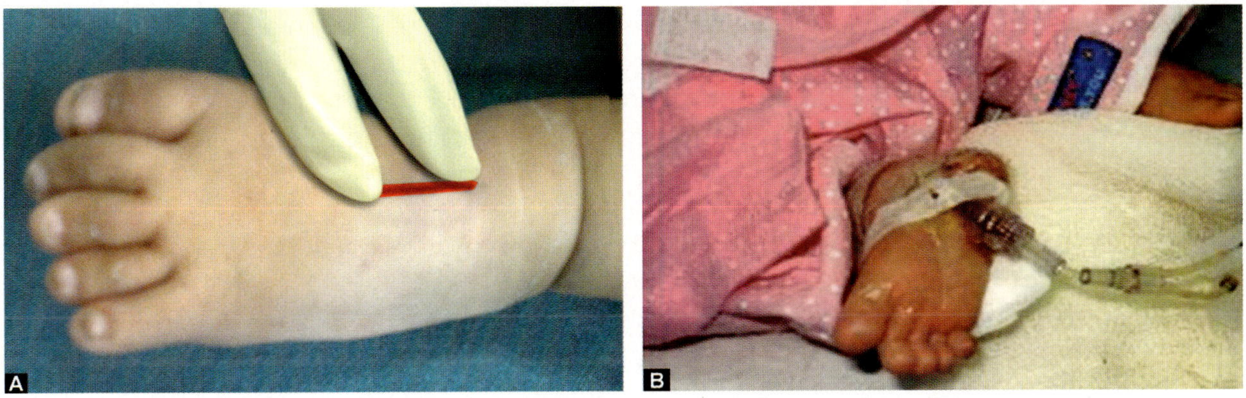

Figs 2.24A and B: (A) Dorsalis pedis artery; (B) Posterior tibial artery cannula *in situ*

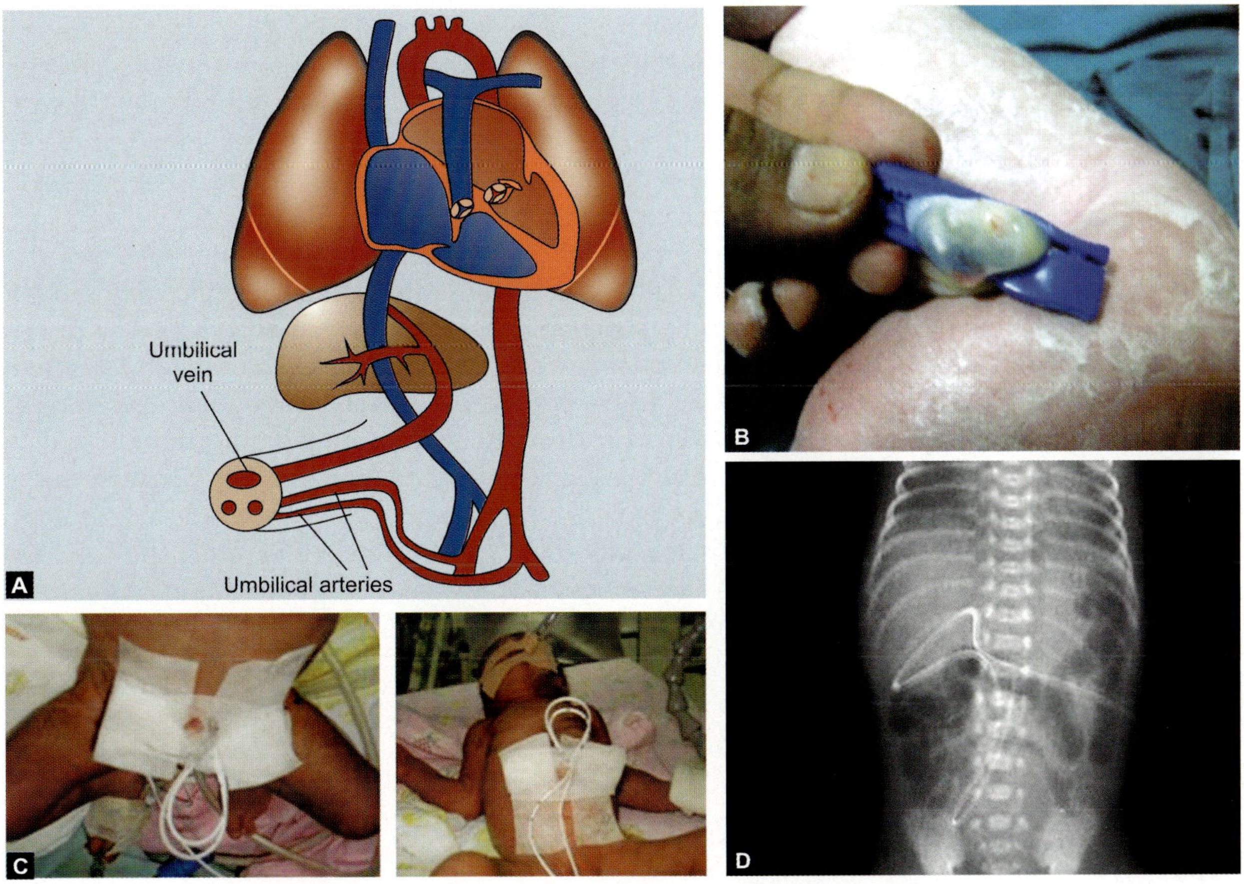

Figs 2.25A to D: (A) Course of umbilical artery; (B) Umbilical artery anatomy; (C) Neonate with UAC and UVC *in situ*; (D) Radiological confirmation

The UAC should be prepared by flushing with a heparin solution (10 units/ml) using a prefilled syringe attached to a 3-way connector. The technique is similar to umbilical vein catheterization up to the step of identification of the vessels. Insert the closed tips of a thin curved forceps into the arterial lumen and dilate the artery. In very low birth weight babies, one tip of the forceps should be enough. Dilating the lumen of the artery is the most important step in UA catheterization, so it should be done gently and patiently. Repeat this several times till the forceps can reach up to its bend. Now insert the catheter tip into the dilated lumen and advance it towards the pelvis. Obstruction may be encountered at level of abdominal wall (<3 cm) or bladder (approximately 5 cm). Gentle and steady pressure for 30-40 seconds is usually enough to overcome the obstruction and stop advancing after reaching the desired distance as given below:

Birth weight (gm)	*Distance for umbilical artery catheter (cm)*
1000	7
1500	8
2000	9
2500	10

Avoid excess pressure to prevent arterial perforation. If obstruction persists, try to cannulate the other artery. Obtain sample and flush with heparinized saline, and avoid bubbles. Secure the catheter with 4-0 silk and connect transducer. Apply antibiotic ointment to the umbilicus, and a dry dressing. Secure the dressing and catheter with tape in a goal-post manner. Seek an alternative site if obstruction persists. Confirm catheter tip radiographically as a malpositioned UAC can have life-threatening consequences. Once the UAC position is verified and hemostasis is maintained, the umbilical tie should be removed.

The tip should be at a high (T_6-T_9) level in the abdominal aorta or at a low level below (L_3-L_4) to ensure catheter is below the origin of the inferior mesenteric and renal arteries. A high-lying line is desirable because chances of limb ischemia are less. Further advancing will pass it through the ductus arteriosus into the pulmonary artery which may lead to errors in treatment as PaO_2 and blood pressure in pulmonary artery are almost always lower than in the aorta. Monitor lower limb perfusion (blanching, mottling, decreased or absent femoral pulse). Warming of opposite limb may help by inducing reflex vasodilation of the affected limb. Document the procedure carefully in the patient's medical record (i.e. catheter type, length inserted, location of tip on X-ray, adjustments made, estimated blood loss, date of insertion, etc.). The UAC can be left in place for 7–10 days, but should be removed at any sign of complication or damping of waveform as these signs are indicative of thrombosis.

Complications

- Thromboembolic events
  - Necrotizing enterocolitis (NEC) due to inferior mesenteric artery thrombosis when the UAC tip is above L_3.
  - Renal artery thrombosis—renal insufficiency, HT
  - Lower limb ischemia, necrosis of digits due to vasospasm
- Blood loss due to accidental disconnection
- Vasospasm, vascular perforation, compartment syndrome
- Infection
- Accidental drug injection
- Aneurysm formation (damage to the arterial wall)
- Hypoglycemia if UAC tip above recommended site. Glucose infusion may stream into the pancreatic artery via the celiac axis, causing hyperinsulinemia and resultant hypoglycemia.

Contraindications

- Omphalitis
- Omphalocele

- Necrotizing enterocolitis
- Peritonitis
- Evidence of vascular compromise in lower limbs.

Caution

- Maintain a constant heparinized (i.e. 1 unit/mL) fluid infusion
- Never infuse pressor agents through a UAC
- Do not feed an infant with UAC and remove the UAC if any sign of NEC
- Samples obtained from UAC are postductal
- During removal, the UAC should be pulled out very slowly @ 1 cm/min for the last 5 cm so as to allow the UA to shrink and go into vasospasm which prevents bleeding.

SETTING UP TRANSDUCER FOR CONTINUOUS PRESSURE MONITORING (FIG. 2.26)

- For continuous monitoring the transducer needs to be placed at the level of the right atrium
- Prime the tubing and transducer with heparinized saline; attach to the cannula
- Attach cable to pressure line on monitor and connect to transducer plug
- Calibrate the transducer to atmosphere
- Ensure continuous/periodic flushing of the system
- Ensure satisfactory waveform
- Strict asepsis should be maintained while handling arterial and venous sites-especially in newborns who are particularly susceptible to nosocomial infections. Regular aseptic dressings and inspection of the site is of prime importance
- The transducer should be leveled correctly at the 4th intercostal space in the midaxillary line
- Accuracy of values depends on the tubing, which should be non-pliant, less than 120 cm in length, should enable transmission of pulsatile impulse from tip of the cannula to the transducer without being compressed and at a similar frequency to the air-fluid interface
- Ensure absence of air bubbles in the tubing
- Screen scale should be adjusted

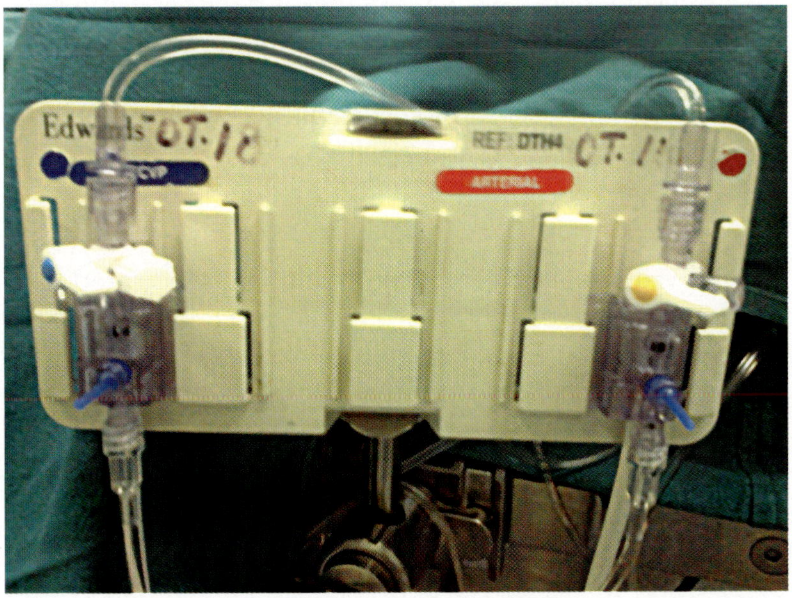

Fig. 2.26: Transducer manifold

- If waveform is present but sample cannot be drawn, it implies that the vessel is in spasm (hypothermia/poor perfusion).

CARE OF THE ARTERIAL LINE

- Suture or tape the arterial line
- Transparent dressing preferred
- Splint the adjoining joint. For radial artery, splint in the semi-dorsiflexed position to prevent kinking
- Infuse heparinized saline 1 ml/hr (0.5–1 unit /ml) to decrease the risk of clotting
- Apply firm pressure at puncture site for 5 minutes after removing cannula
- Ensure that fingers and toes are visible.

REMOVING THE ARTERIAL LINE

- Stop infusion of heparinized saline just before removing arterial line
- Remove the overlying dressing while palpating the artery
- Withdraw the catheter slowly; compress the puncture site for 3-5 minutes
- Continue checking the limb perfusion
- Check for hematoma and bleeding
- Never put a compression dressing over the insertion site.

Intraosseous Vascular Access

Intraosseous (IO) infusion is an effective, reliable and relatively simple technique, both for obtaining rapid vascular access and for the administration of fluids and medications in the emergency setting.

Placing an intravenous access in an adult in a moving ambulance can take 10-12 minutes, with a 10-40% failure rate while there is 70-100% success rate for pediatric and adult intraosseous needle placement, often within one minute.

In shock, blood is shunted to the "core" organs, namely the heart, lungs and brain, and away from the periphery. This "diving reflex" mechanism makes peripheral intravenous access difficult even in the most skilled hands. In contrast to the peripheral vasculature, the intraosseous space—a rich network of blood vessels within the bone-remains unchanged by the effects of shock. The bone marrow functions as a "non-collapsible" vein and is able to provide a route for rapid vascular access in infants, children and adults.

INDICATION

Intraosseous infusion is a viable option for any age group. It is indicated in infants and children of any age where peripheral IV appears to be difficult or has been unsuccessful (90 seconds, three attempts or whichever comes first). Recent technological advances have made IO devices a viable and reliable alternative to traditional adult IV access. A practical approach is to pursue IO and peripheral or central venous access simultaneously.

ACCESS SITES

The most common site recommended is the proximal tibia because it provides a flat surface with a thin layer of overlying tissue and ease of identifying landmarks. Also, it is distant from the airway and chest, where resuscitation attempts are in progress. The other sites are distal

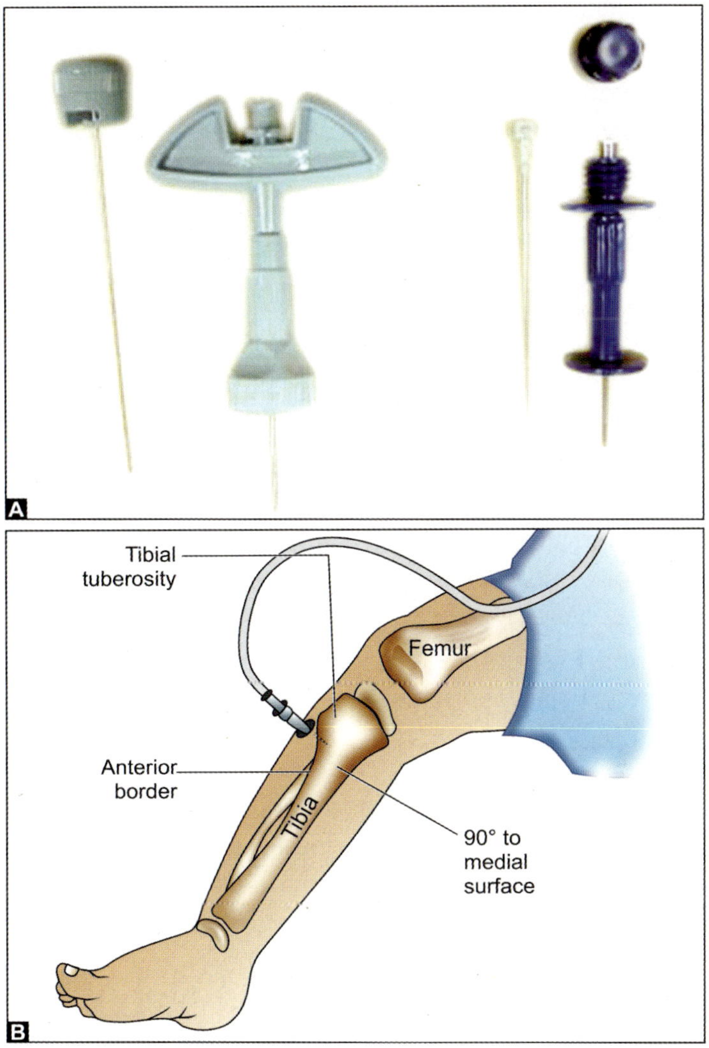

Figs 2.27A and B: (A) IO needle; (B) IO technique

tibia (1-2 cm proximal to the medial malleolus of tibia) and lower third of femur (3 cm above lateral condyle in the midline). So whichever site is chosen, it should be easily accessible and should not interfere with procedures like spinal immobilization or CPR.

PROCEDURE

The ideal device or needle should be small, lightweight, reloadable, inexpensive and easily inserted under any condition. Spinal or hypodermic needles are usually not suitable since they are available in narrow gauge and tend to bend and do not provide good hand grip **(Figs 2.27A and B)**:

- Identify the tibial tuberosity just below the knee by palpation
- Locate a consistent flat area of bone 2 cm distal and slightly medial to the tibial tuberosity. (Identifying these landmarks helps in avoiding the growth plate)
- Support the flexed knee by placing a towel under the calf
- If time permits, cleanse the area with iodine solution and drape it. Perform insertion using sterile gloves
- Inject local anesthetic (1% lidocaine) into the skin, into the subcutaneous tissue and over the periosteum, especially if the patient is awake

- Insert the IO needle through the skin and subcutaneous tissue; this should be possible with no hindrance. Upon reaching the bone, hold the needle with the index finger and thumb as close to the entry point as possible and with constant pressure on the needle with the palm of the same hand, use a twisting motion to advance the needle through the cortex into the marrow. A 10-15° caudal angulation may be used to further decrease the risk of puncturing the growth plate, but direct entry parallel to the bone is acceptable
- Advance the needle from the cortex into the marrow space, at which point a popping sensation or lack of resistance is felt. Do not advance the needle any further
- The first indication of proper placement occurs when the needle stands up on its own. At this point, remove the inner trocar, attach a 5 ml syringe to the needle, and aspirate bone marrow. Obtaining marrow confirms placement
- If marrow is not aspirated, push a 5 to 10 ml bolus of isotonic sodium chloride solution through the syringe. Resistance to flow should be minimal and extravasation should not be evident. Observing the calf area for extravasation is important
- If flow is good and extravasation is not evident, connect an intravenous line with a 3-way stopcock to the needle, and secure the needle with gauze pads and tape
- Restrain the leg and maintain a clean infusion site while the needle is in place.

Though most commonly left in place for a few hours (3-4 hr), some IOs have been in place for as long as 24 hours without sequelae.

POTENTIAL COMPLICATIONS

- Extravasation of fluids and medications and compartment syndrome: Regular checks of the insertion site is essential and remove IO needle if this complication is suspected. Do not insert a new IO in the same bone.
- Hematoma formation
- Micro fat embolism
- Osteomyelitis, subcutaneous abscess, bacteremia
- Growth plate injury (with incorrect placement)

EFFECTIVENESS OF IO VERSUS IV ACCESS

When an IO needle is correctly placed, fluid and medications can be administered just as if an IV line was in place **(Table 2.4)**. The intraosseous space is a specialized area of the vascular

Table 2.4: Fluids and drugs that can be given through intraosseous route

Anesthetics	*Resuscitation drugs*	*Fluids*	*Neuromuscular blockers*	*Anticonvulsants*
Propofol	Lidocaine	NS, RL, DNS	Pancuronium	Phenobarbitone
Ketamine	Epinephrine	Blood	Vecuronium	Phenytoin
Thiopentone sodium	Dopamine	Plasma	Atracurium	Diazepam
	Dobutamine	Hypertonic saline	Succinylcholine	Morphine
	Atropine	Dextrose		Fentanyl
	Digoxin			
	Sodium bicarbonate			
	Calcium chloride			
	Calcium gluconate			
	Adenosine			

system. Resting pressure in the intraosseous space (10-35 mm Hg) is generally a value between mean arterial pressure (50-100 mm Hg) and venous pressure (0-10 mm Hg). Though fluid may flow due to gravity into an IO line, the flow rate for bolus infusions can be optimized if a syringe or pressure bag (inflated up to 300 mm Hg) is used. Utilizing these methods, flow rates in excess of 40 cc/min (2400 cc/hr) can be achieved, and a pediatric 20 cc/kg fluid bolus can be given over 5-6 minutes.

Though its use has declined with advent of newer intravenous catheters and alternative access techniques, it still has a major role in life-threatening emergency situations when other accesses fail and time is of utmost importance.

3 Pain Management

As the practice of anesthesiology extends itself beyond perioperative medicine, the anesthesiologist's knowledge and expertise in pain assessment and management is highly valued. There is growing evidence that pediatric patients of all ages, even the extremely premature neonates, are capable of experiencing pain as a result of tissue injuries due to various causes.

There are several physiological consequences and behavioral responses of pain in children and therefore they need to be addressed **(Table 3.1)**.

Table 3.1: Physiological consequences of pain in children

Increased blood pressure	Increased O_2 consumption
Increased heart rate	Decreased tidal volume
Hypermetabolism	Decreased FRC
Hyperglycemia	V/Q mismatch
Protein catabolism	Decreased cough
Lipolysis	Decreased gut motility
Increased cardiac output	Sodium and water retention
Hypercoagulability	Altered immune function
Increased fibrinolysis	

Assessment of Pain

Pain is a subjective experience, so assessment of degree of pain remains a challenging task in children because of communication barrier. Pain assessment is the first step in management of pain. The Joint Commission of Accreditation of Health Care Organization (JCAHO) considers pain to be the fifth vital sign.

Apart from physiological response to pain, several pain measurement tools can be broadly classified into behavioral measures, composite measures and self report **(Table 3.2)**.

PHYSIOLOGICAL PARAMETERS

Increase in heart rate, respiratory rate, blood pressure and palmar sweating are some of the physiological measures used to measure pain. These parameters may be influenced by factors like hypoxemia, hypovolemia, and fever which are unrelated to pain.

Table 3.2: Pain assessment method

Age-group	*Self-report*	*Behavioral*	*Composite*
Preverbal (Neonates and infants)		NIPS FLACC	PIPP* **(Table 3.3)** CRIES COMFORT
Pre-schoolers	FACES pain scale* **(Figs 3.1A and B)** Poker chip tool Ladder scale Eland color scale	FLACC CHEOPS	OPS COMFORT
Schoolers	VAS* **(Fig. 3.2)** NRS – 11, 101 Modified McGill pain questionnaire		COMFORT

* The most commonly used scale in each group is described below

Table 3.3: Premature infant pain profile (PIPP)

Indicators	*Score* 0	1	2	3
Gestational age	≥ 36 weeks	32–35+6 weeks	28–31+6 weeks	< 28 weeks
Behavioral state before pain stimulus (observe for 15 sec)	Active/awake Eyes open Facial movement	Quiet/awake Eyes open No facial movement	Active/sleep Eyes closed Facial movement	Quiet/sleep Eyes closed No facial movement
During painful stimulus				
Change in HR	↑ 0-4 bpm	↑ 5-14 bpm	↑ 15-24 bpm	↑ ≥ 25 bpm
Change in SaO_2	↓ 0-2.4%	↓ 2.5-4.9%	↓ 5-7.4%	↓ ≥ 7.5%
Brow bulge	None ≤ 9% of time	Minimal 10-39%	Moderate 40-69%	Maximum ≥ 70%
Eye squeeze	None ≤ 9% of time	Minimal 10-39%	Moderate 40-69%	Maximum ≥ 70%
Nasolabial furrow	None ≤ 9% of time	Minimal 10-39%	Moderate 40-69%	Maximum ≥ 70%

- Score = 0-21
- Higher the score, the greater is the pain behavior

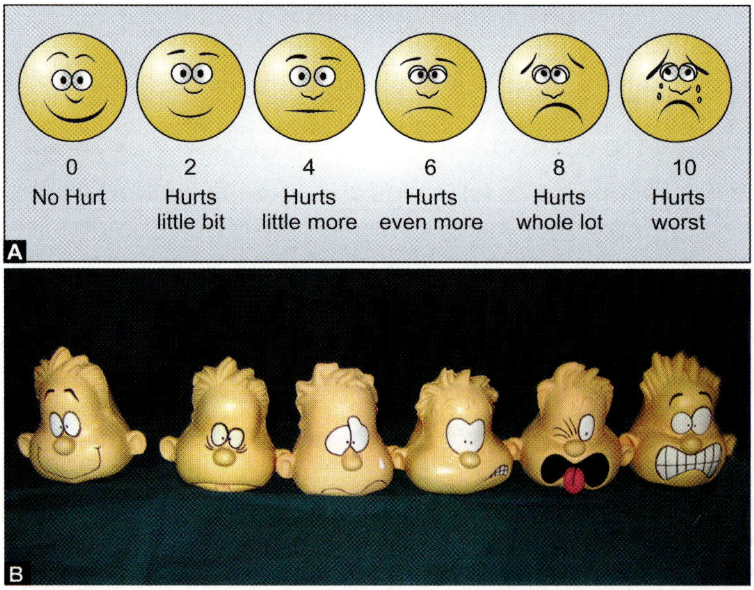

Figs 3.1A and B: (A) Faces Pain Scale (The Wong Baker Scale); (B) Face models for pain assessment in PACU

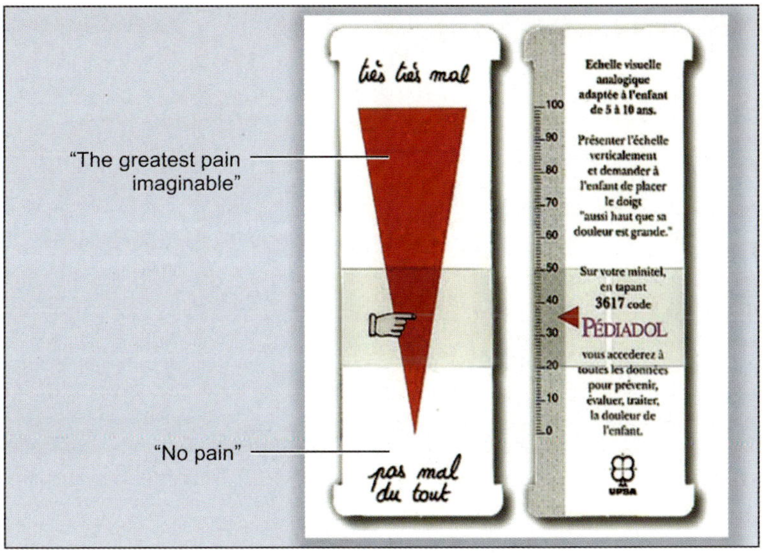

Fig. 3.2: Visual analog scale (VAS)
It is unidimensional and measures only intensity of pain
0 = no pain
10 = worst pain imaginable

BEHAVIORAL MEASURES

Changes in facial expression, movement of torso and limbs, type of cry, consolability and sleep state are some of the behavioral changes seen in response to pain in young children.

COMPOSITE MEASURES

Scales like COMFORT, CHEOPS and FLACC are more comprehensive as they include both physiological and behavioral changes in determining pain scores. The scale used in the assessment of pain depends on the age group of the child.

SELF REPORT

Self report may be considered the gold standard in children and is usually possible by 2-4 years of age. Children may cooperate in using *Faces Pain Scale* and may grade pain if trained properly.

Management of Postoperative Pain

Classification of pain as acute or chronic defines the approach to treatment with immediate and aggressive treatment of acute pain and a planned multimodal approach to chronic pain.

Pain management plans which target multiple steps in the complex nociceptive process by using a combination of analgesics are more effective than plans that target a single step. The various analgesics and techniques used to treat acute pain in children are as follows:

1. Simple analgesics, e.g. paracetamol **(Table 3.4, Fig. 3.3A)**
2. NSAIDs, e.g. ibuprofen, diclofenac, ketorolac, etc. **(Table 3.5, Fig. 3.3B)**
3. Narcotics—morphine, fentanyl, tramadol, etc. **(Table 3.6)**
4. Local anesthetics (topical, infiltration, regional blocks).

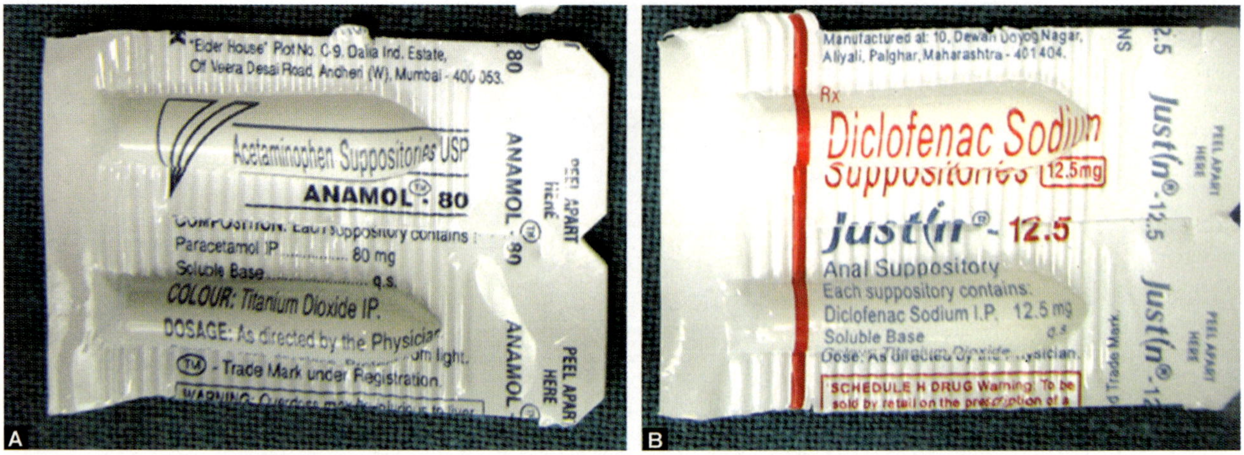

Figs 3.3A and B: (A) Paracetamol suppository; (B) Diclofenac suppository

Table 3.4: Paracetamol dosing guide

Age	*Maximum daily dose (mg kg^{-1})*		*IV infusion over 15 min (mg kg^{-1})*	*Rectal dose (mg kg^{-1})*		*Oral (mg kg^{-1})*
	Oral/Rectal	*Intravenous*		*Repeat*	*Single*	
28–32 weeks	40	30	7.5	20	35-45	10-15
32–38 weeks	60		4-6 hrly	12 hrly		4-6 hrly
Infants	75	60	15	20		
Children	100*		4-6 hrly	6 hrly		

* maximum up to 4 gm

Table 3.5: Dose of NSAIDs*

Drug	*Route*	*Dose*	*Maximum daily dose*
Diclofenac	Oral/rectal	1 mg kg^{-1} (maximum dose 50 mg) 8 hrly	150 mg day^{-1}
Ibuprofen	Oral	10 mg kg^{-1} 6 hrly	40 mg kg^{-1} day^{-1}
Ketorolac	Oral	0.25 mg kg^{-1}	1 mg kg^{-1} day^{-1} (maximum for 7 days)
	Intravenous	0.5–1 mg kg^{-1}	30 mg day^{-1} (maximum for 5 days)

* The above NSAIDs are not indicated in infants less than six months of age and children with asthma, renal impairment or bleeding disorders

Usually narcotics like morphine and fentanyl are administered as IV or IM bolus, but if the hospital has adequate facility with trained nurses for 'nurse controlled analgesia,' these drugs can be given as continuous infusion via infusion pump or patient controlled analgesia (PCA) pump.

Table 3.6: Dose of IV narcotics							
Drug	*Bolus ($\mu g\ kg^{-1}$)*	*Infusion* ($\mu g\ kg^{-1}\ hr^{-1}$)*	*PCA**				
			Demand ($\mu g\ kg^{-1}$)	*LOI (min)*	*Basal ($\mu g\ kg^{-1}\ hr^{-1}$)*	*1 hr/4 hr limit ($\mu g\ kg^{-1}$)*	*Rescue IV dose ($\mu g\ kg^{-1}$)*
Morphine							
• Preterm	10-25 2-4 hrly	2-5	20	8-10	0-20	100/300	50
• Full term	25-50 3-4 hrly	5-10					
• Infants and children	50-100 3-4 hrly	15-30					
Fentanyl	0.5-1 1-2 hrly	0.5	0.5	6-8	0-0.5	2.5/4	0.5-1
Remifentanil	1-2	3-10					
Tramadol	1-2 mg kg^{-1}	0.5-1 mg $kg^{-1}\ hr^{-1}$					

* Preparation of infusion → Morphine: 1 mg kg^{-1} in 50 ml diluent (1 ml = 20 $\mu g\ kg^{-1}$)
Fentanyl: 25 $\mu g\ kg^{-1}$ in 50 ml diluent (1 ml = 0.5 $\mu g\ kg^{-1}$)

Topical Analgesia

EUTECTIC MIXTURE OF LOCAL ANESTHETICS (EMLA) (FIG. 3.4)

Indications

Minor procedures such as venipuncture, circumcision, lumbar puncture, arterial cannulation, etc.

EMLA is an oil in water emulsion of 2.5% lidocaine and 2.5% prilocaine achieving 80% of drug in active unchanged (base) form. Application of a thick layer of cream over intact skin

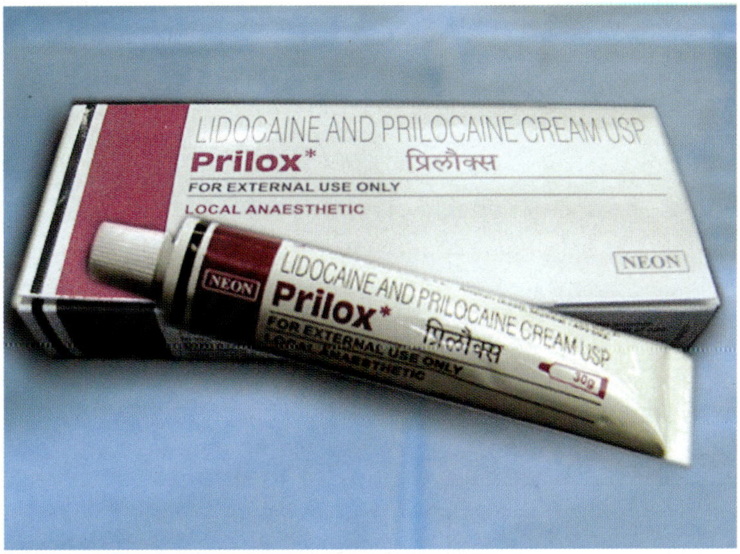

Fig. 3.4: EMLA cream

covered with an occlusive dressing for 45 minutes to 1 hour gives 1–2 hours of analgesia after removal. Application of an external heat pack can reduce onset time to 20 minutes. Caution is to be exercised in premature babies due to methemoglobinemia risk from prilocaine.

Contraindications

- Allergy to local anesthetics
- Broken skin
- Congenital or acquired methemoglobinemia.

Wound Irrigation

Anesthetic solutions like TAC (Tetracaine 0.5%–Adrenaline–1:4000-Cocaine 4%) and LET (Lidocaine–Epinephrine–Tetracaine) is administered by a swab pressed firmly to a wound in a dose of 3-5 ml/3 cm of laceration. These solutions do not work on intact skin but are effective in lacerations within 10-20 minutes. Since LET contains epinephrine, it should not be applied to areas supplied by end arteries.

Wound Infiltration

0.25% plain bupivacaine, up to 0.5 ml/kg is used for wound infiltration either before or at the end of the procedure **(Fig. 3.5)**. Aspirate frequently to avoid accidental intravascular injection and avoid infiltration into muscle as this will result in high blood level. Wound infiltration reduces opioid requirement.

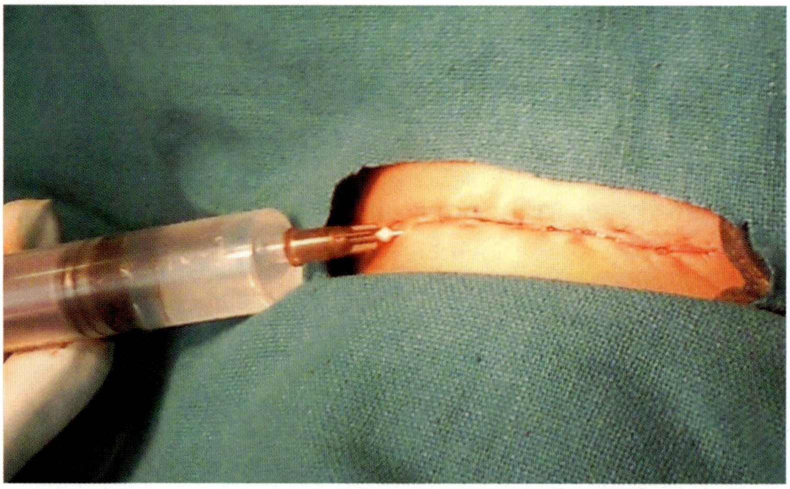

Fig. 3.5: Wound infiltration

Regional Analgesia Techniques

In present day practice, pediatric anesthesiologists view regional anesthesia as an adjunct to general anesthesia.

A better knowledge of the pharmacokinetics of local anesthetics in infants and children along with the development of regional anesthesia techniques with availability of better equipment specially designed for children has allowed the implementation of safe and effective regional blocks in this age group.

COMMON PRINCIPLES FOR A SAFE AND EFFECTIVE BLOCK

1. A clear understanding of the differences in anatomy, physiology and drug pharmacokinetics from adults while performing blocks is essential.
2. General anesthesia is necessary in most children for performing regional blocks except in ex-premature babies.
3. Only short beveled needles should be used for blocks for better appreciation of the loss of resistance while piercing fascia and aponeurosis.
4. Injection of local anesthetic should never be attempted if there is resistance. This is the best way of preventing neural damage.
5. Ultrasound guided block techniques may be safer and superior to blind techniques which rely on subtle sensation that may be unreliable even in experienced hands.
6. In case of surgery of short duration, the patient requires vigilance and monitoring beyond the time to peak blood concentration of the local anesthetic.

Neuraxial Block

Significant anatomical differences exist between children and adults in view of neuraxial block (Fig. 3.6):

1. The conus medullaris ends at the L_3 vertebra in neonates and infants compared to the L_1 vertebra in adults. So dural puncture below L_3-L_4 is advised in neonates and infants.
2. The dural sac ends at S_3-S_4 vertebrae in neonates and infants compared to S_1-S_2 in small children and adults, so inadvertent dural puncture is a possibility during caudal block in infants.
3. Tuffier's line (intercristal line that stretches across the top of both iliac crests) crosses the L_5–S_1 interspace in neonates, L_4-L_5 interspace in infants and small children as compared to L_4 vertebra in adults. So this line remains the landmark for dural puncture in all age groups.
4. The sacrum in children is flat, narrow, partly cartilaginous, more cephalad and easily palpated, due to absence of fat over it in comparison to adults. Therefore, caudal block is easier in children than in adults. Intraosseous injection also remains a possibility in small children.

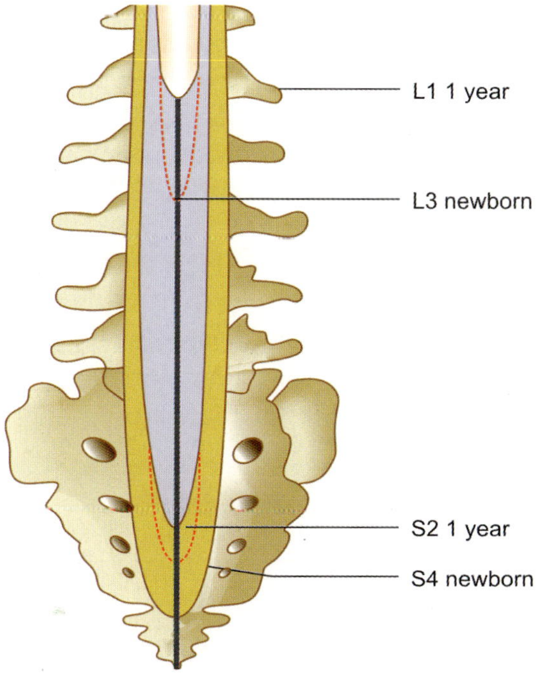

Fig. 3.6: Difference in neuraxial anatomy

5. Contents of the epidural space are more gelatinous and less fibrous until 7–8 years of age in comparison to the densely packed fat lobules divided by fibrous strands in adults. So advancement of epidural catheter as well as spread of local anesthetics is easier in children less than 8 years of age.
6. In an infant, the nerve fiber diameter is smaller with thinner myelin sheath and smaller internodal distance, so a lower concentration of local anesthetic, but larger volume is needed to cover multiple dermatomes.

PHYSIOLOGY AND DRUG PHARMACOKINETICS IN THE PEDIATRIC AGE GROUP

1. In children less than eight years of age, hemodynamic instability is not seen with the sympathectomy associated with neuraxial block. This is possibly due to a lower resting sympathetic control over vascular tone in children as well as a greater ability to compensate for decrease in systemic vascular resistance. So preloading is not required even with high spinal block in children.
2. Children respond differently to local anesthetics because of an immature hepatic enzyme system with decreased hepatic blood flow, reduced plasma cholinesterase levels, increased volume of distribution and reduced level of albumin and alpha-1 glycoprotein. In neonates and infants, local anesthetic toxicity may result from the increased plasma levels of free drug due to decreased protein binding and decreased drug clearance because of low level of cytochrome P450, especially in the scenario of higher dose or prolonged infusion. Thus, the maximum dose of local anesthetics should be decreased by 50% in infants less than six months of age **(Table 3.7)**.

Table 3.7: Maximum allowable dosing guidelines

Local anesthetic	*Single dose (mg kg^{-1})*		*Continuous infusion rate (mg kg^{-1} hr^{-1})*	
	Neonates	*Children*	*Neonates*	*Children*
Bupivacaine	2	3	0.2	0.4
Levobupivacaine	2	3	0.2	0.4
Ropivacaine	2	3	0.2	0.4
Lidocaine	5		1.0	1.5
Lidocaine with epinephrine	7		NR	NR

NR – not recommended

3. CSF volume in infants and newborns is 4 ml/kg in comparison to 2 ml/kg in adults. The larger CSF volume per body weight basis accounts for higher dose and shorter duration of action of local anesthetics in subarachnoid block in infants.
4. Cardiotoxicity of racemic bupivacaine is predominantly due to the dextroisomer, the levoisomer of bupivacaine is equipotent with a higher safety profile.
5. Neonates may have immature ventilatory responses to hypoxia and hypercarbia and so are at a greater risk for respiratory depression in case of overdosage with narcotics.

Epidural Analgesia

Method	**Approach**
Single shot technique	Caudal/lumbar
Catheter technique	
Intermittent bolus	Caudal lumbar Caudal thoracic Lumbar epidural
Continuous infusion	Lumbar thoracic Thoracic epidural

CURRENT TREND OF ADJUVANTS USED IN EPIDURAL SPACE

Various adjuvants may be used to prolong the duration of blockade particularly for the single-shot technique.

- *Epinephrine* was the most commonly used in concentration of 1:200,000 (5 μg/ml^{-1}) to 1: 400,000 (2.5 μg/ml), but not preferred now due to the theoretical disadvantage of potential spinal cord ischemia secondary to impaired blood flow to the artery of Adamkiewicz.

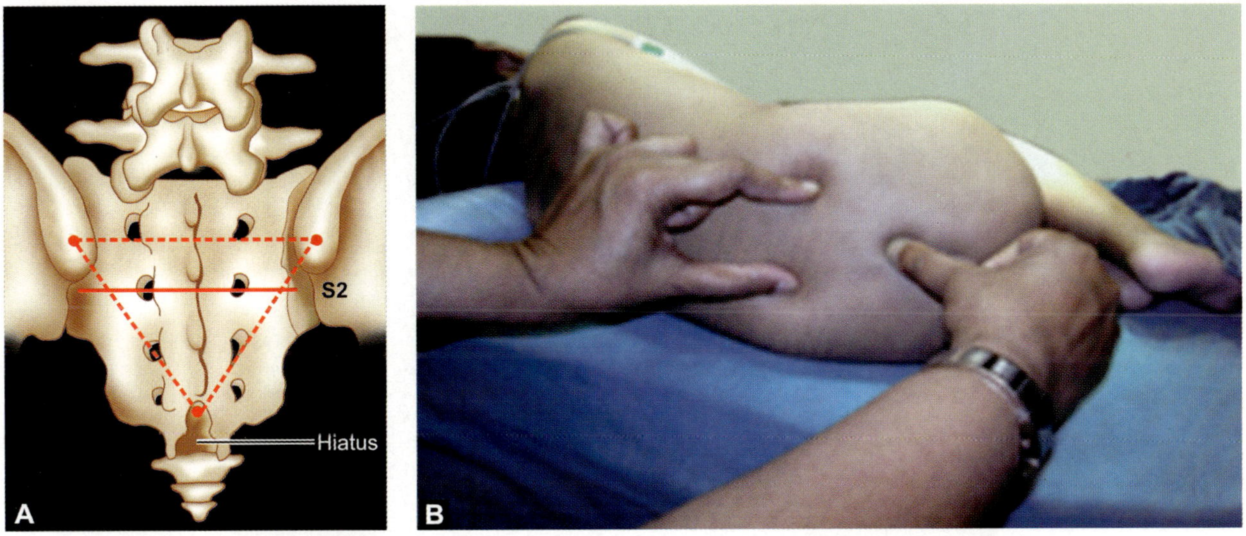

Figs 3.7A and B: (A) Sacral anatomy; (B) Surface landmarks for caudal block

- *Opioids* are used judiciously in ambulatory cases because of side effects like nausea, vomiting, itching, urine retention and respiratory depression.
- *Clonidine* potentiates analgesia and prolongs duration without side-effects. A dose of 1-2 µg/kg is used for single shot caudal block and 0.1 µg/kg/hr for an epidural infusion.
- *Ketamine* in a low dose (0.25–0.5 mg/kg) prolongs analgesia without psychomimetic effects.
- *Midazolam* in a dose of 50 µg/kg produces analgesia without behavioral changes or motor weakness.
- *Neostigmine* is unsuitable for day care surgery due to a high incidence of emesis.

SINGLE-SHOT CAUDAL EPIDURAL (FIGS 3.7A AND B)

- Most commonly used regional block in children.
- Indicated in surgery below umbilicus (T_{10} dermatome)
- Demerits are short duration of action and limited dermatomal distribution.

Technique

After induction of GA, the sacral hiatus is palpated with the patient in lateral position. The sacral hiatus is formed by non fusion of the S_5 vertebral arch and lies at the apex of an equilateral triangle, the base of which is formed by the line joining the two posterosuperior iliac spines. A 22G or 23 G hypodermic needle is inserted at the apex of the hiatus at 70° angle to the skin until a classic 'pop' is felt with penetration of the sacrococcygeal ligament. The needle is then advanced a further 2 mm more into the sacral canal and stabilized with the left hand. After negative aspiration for blood or CSF, the local anesthetic is slowly injected while monitoring the ECG for any change in heart rate, rhythm or amplitude **(Fig. 3.8)** **(Table 3.8)**. In case of bloody tap, the needle is removed and the whole process is repeated.

Table 3.8: Dosage of LA for caudal block

Volume	*Segment*	*Concentration*	*Total dose*
0.5 ml /kg	Sacral	≤ 0.2% ropivacaine	
0.75 ml/kg	L_1	≤ 0.25% bupivacaine	not exceeding total allowable dose
1.0 ml/kg	T_{10}		
1.25 ml/kg	T_6		

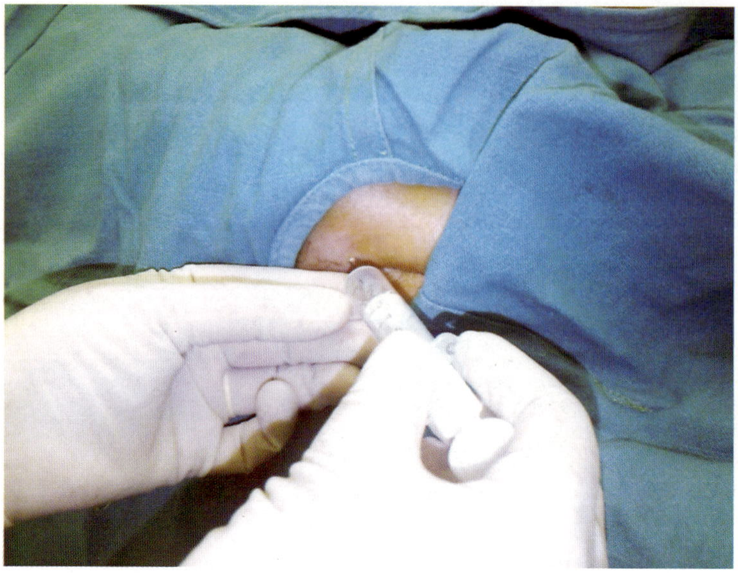

Fig. 3.8: Caudal epidural block

THREADING A CAUDAL EPIDURAL CATHETER TO LUMBAR/THORACIC SPACE

An epidural catheter is inserted through 19–20 G Tuohy needle inserted in sacral hiatus by the technique of a single shot approach. The appropriate length of catheter to be left inside the epidural space should be measured against the back of the child from the puncture site to the target spinal level. Minor resistance to the passage of the catheter can be overcome by flexion or extension of the spine, using a styletted catheter, epidural stimulation technique, etc. Caudal epidural catheters are usually restricted to 48 hours for fear of contamination from the perineal area.

Indications

Useful for surgery involving dermatomes above T_{10} level.

Advantage

Less risk of dural puncture or spinal cord trauma than a direct thoracic epidural approach.

Confirmation of Epidural Catheter Tip

1. X-ray imaging with contrast or radiopaque catheter
2. Fluoroscopy real-time imaging while placing the catheter
3. Epidural electrical stimulation causes muscles to twitch in the lower limbs, followed by the abdominal muscles and finally the intercostal muscles as the epidural catheter is advanced
4. Epidural ECG—compares ECG signal from the tip of catheter with the signal from a surface electrode at target segmental level.

LUMBAR EPIDURAL BLOCK

Usually a continuous catheter technique.

Indications

Long-term analgesia after major thoracic, abdominal or lower extremity surgical procedures.

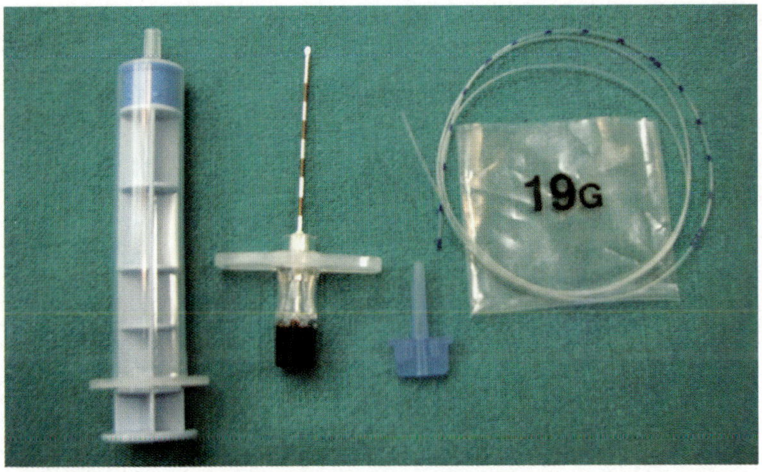

Fig. 3.9: Pediatric epidural set

Technique

Similar to that in adult but with a few differences:

1. Appropriate size of needle and catheter is important. An 18G (10 cm) Tuohy needle with 20G catheter for more than five years of age and 19G (5 cm) Tuohy needle with 19 G epidural catheter for less than 5 years of age **(Fig. 3.9)**. A very thin catheter frequently triggers the infusion alarm system due to resistance.
2. Distance from skin to epidural space is shallow.
   Mean depth in neonates is 1 cm
   Formulae for rough guideline for depth of needle insertion:
   Rough estimate = 1 mm/kg body weight
   Depth (cm) = 1 + 0.15 × age (years)
   Depth (cm) = 0.8 + 0.05 × weight (kg)
3. Epidural space location is done by loss of resistance (LOR) technique with saline to reduce the risk of venous air embolism, cord compression or a patchy block in neonates and infants **(Fig. 3.10)**.

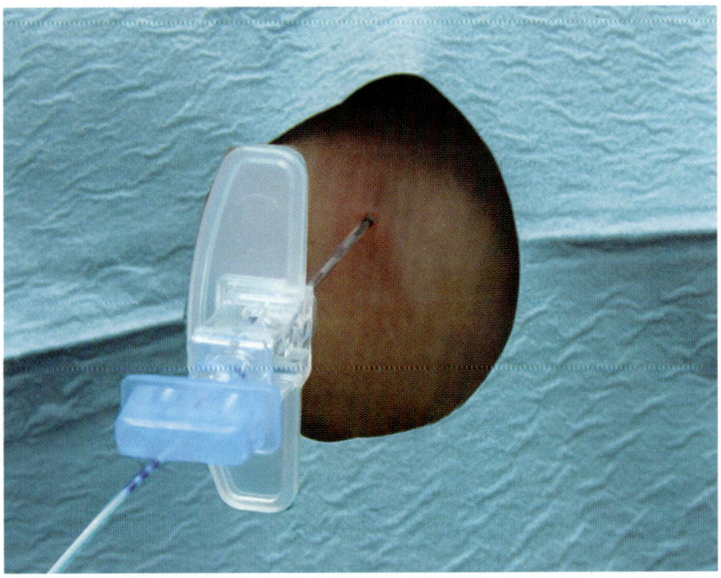

Fig. 3.10: Epidural injection

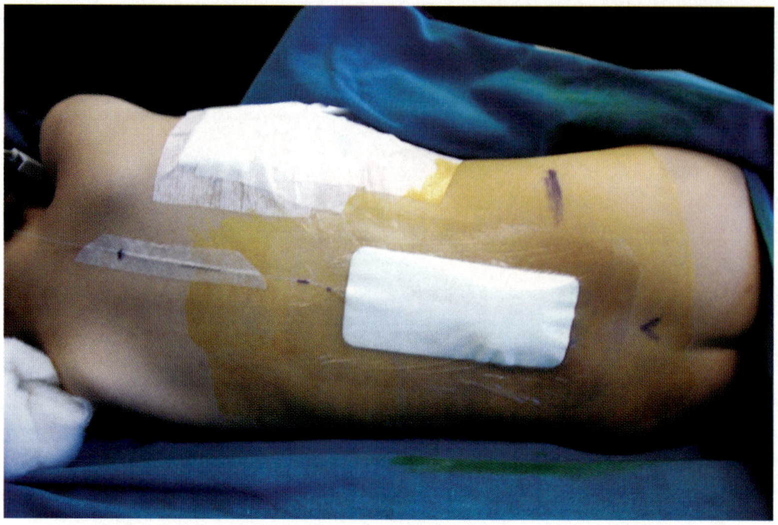

Fig. 3.11: Transparent dressing of epidural catheter

4. A distinct 'pop' may not be felt while penetrating the less tensile ligamentum flavum in infants, so rapid advancement of needle should be avoided to prevent dural puncture.
5. After negative aspiration and subsequent test dosing, the target dose is injected slowly (0.5 ml/min) in infants. The test dose consists of 0.5 μg/kg of epinephrine or 0.1 ml/kg of local anesthetic with epinephrine (1:200000) **(Table 3.9)**.
6. An epidural catheter dislodges very easily in children. It should be secured well with transparent adhesive dressing **(Fig. 3.11)**.
7. The length of catheter in the epidural space is according to the patient's length and target dermatome.

Table 3.9: Dosage of bupivacaine for epidural block

Approach	*Concentration*	*Age*		*Fentanyl*
		< 6 months	*> 6 months*	
Lumbar				
• Bolus	0.25%	0.3 ml kg^{-1}	0.5 ml kg^{-1}	1-3 μg kg^{-1}
• Top-up (after 90 min)	0.25%	0.15 ml kg^{-1}	0.25 ml kg^{-1}	
• More injections (after same interval)	0.25%	half of second dose	half of second dose	
Lumbar infusion	0.125%	0.2 mg kg^{-1} hr^{-1}	0.4 mg kg^{-1} hr^{-1}	
Thoracic infusion	0.125%	0.1 mg kg^{-1} hr^{-1}	0.2 mg kg^{-1} hr^{-1}	
PCEA >5 years **(Fig. 3.12)**	0.125%	Basal infusion = 0.1-0.2 ml kg^{-1} hr^{-1} Demand dose = 0.05-0.1 ml kg^{-1} LOI = 20-30 minutes Total dose = 0.2-0.4 ml kg^{-1} hr^{-1} Total hourly dose not to exceed 20 ml		

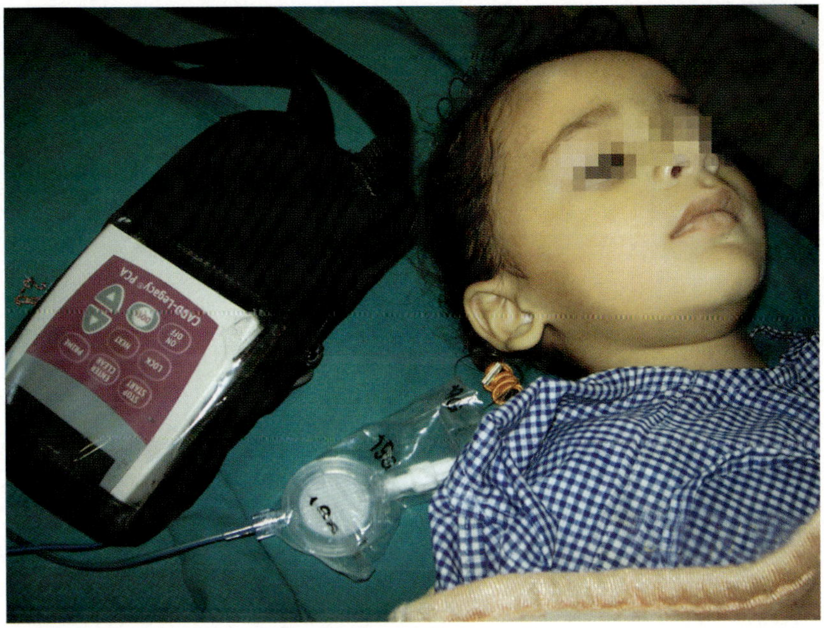

Fig. 3.12: Epidural PCA

THORACIC EPIDURAL ANALGESIA

Indication

Extensive thoracic and abdominal surgical procedures.

Key Points

1. Thoracic epidural is to be performed only by skilled practitioners at tertiary centers.
2. This procedure shoulder be done only in older children as threading a thoracic catheter from the lumbar or caudal route is not possible.
3. The procedure is done under heavy sedation or GA using the electrical stimulation test for safety.

Disadvantage

Possible direct needle trauma to the spinal cord as there are no warning signs under sedation/GA.

Technique

1. Midline approach—lower border of scapula is the anatomical landmark.
2. Epidural needle is inserted in a cephalad direction at 70 degrees angle to the longitudinal axis of the spine. The rest is same as in the lumbar technique.
3. Lower thoracic (T_{10}–T_{12}) approach is easier than mid thoracic (T_4–T_7) level.
4. Rough guideline for estimating skin-epidural distance in children:
   a. 2.15 + (0.01 × age in months) in cm
   b. 1.95 + (0.045 × weight in kg) in cm.

Ropivacaine and 2-chloroprocaine are preferred in neonates. 2-chloroprocaine avoids the potential toxicity of amides because plasma esterase activity, though measurably reduced in

Table 3.10: Continuous epidural dosing guidelines for ropivacaine

Age	*Ropivacaine (µg/ml)*	*Fentanyl (µg/ml)*	*Morphine (µg/ml)*	*Clonidine (µg/ml)*	*Rate of ropivacaine Max (mg/kg/h)*
0-2 months	0.5–1	0.2	NR	0.04	0.2 (0.15-0.25)
Infant	0.5-1.5	1-2	25	0.4	0.25 (0.15-0.3)
Child (lumbar)	1-2	2-4	25-50	0.4-0.6	0.3 (0.2-0.4)
Child (thoracic)	1-2	2-4	NR	0.4-0.6	0.3 (0.2-0.4)
PCEA >5 years	Basal = 0.1-0.2 ml kg^{-1} hr^{-1} Demand = 0.05-0.1 ml kg^{-1} LOI = 20-30 min Total dose = 0.2-0.4 ml kg^{-1} hr^{-1} (not to exceed >20 ml hr^{-1})			Same concentration as above according to age	

neonates, is sufficient for ester metabolism. Ropivacaine is preferred to bupivacaine because its equipotent analgesic dose causes less motor blockade, has a larger therapeutic window and less toxicity. The toxicity is not influenced by duration of infusion for up to 48 to 72 hours in neonates **(Table 3.10)**.

Subarachnoid Block

INDICATIONS

Premature or ex-premature infants undergoing lower abdominal surgery of less than 90 minutes duration.

TECHNIQUE

1. Topical EMLA application at puncture site one hour prior to block.
2. OT should be warm and quiet.
3. Standard monitoring devices (ECG, NIBP, and SpO_2) applied prior to block.
4. Position—lateral decubitus or sitting. Avoid neck flexion as it may cause airway occlusion.
5. Sterile preparation with povidone iodine.
6. Tuffier's line is the anatomical landmark and midline approach is preferred (L_4-L_5 / L_5-S_1).
7. Hypodermic needle 22G (2.5 cm) or 25G (1.5 cm) spinal needle with stylet is used **(Fig. 3.13A)**.
8. The average distance from skin to subarachnoid space is 1 to 1.5 cm.
9. Once free flow of CSF occurs, local anesthetic is injected slowly. If no CSF flow occurs even after apparent correct placement of needle in lateral position, sitting position may be tried **(Fig. 3.13B)**.
10. The ligamentum flavum is very soft in small children and may not allow a "pop" feeling with dural penetration, so frequent withdrawal of stylet may be required to detect subarachnoid space.

DOSAGE

There is a fairly wide therapeutic range in dose of local anesthetic in infants **(Table 3.11)**.

Remember to add the volume of dead space of the spinal needle (0.05–0.1 ml) to the calculated volume of local anesthetic. The prolonged half-lives of bupivacaine and tetracaine

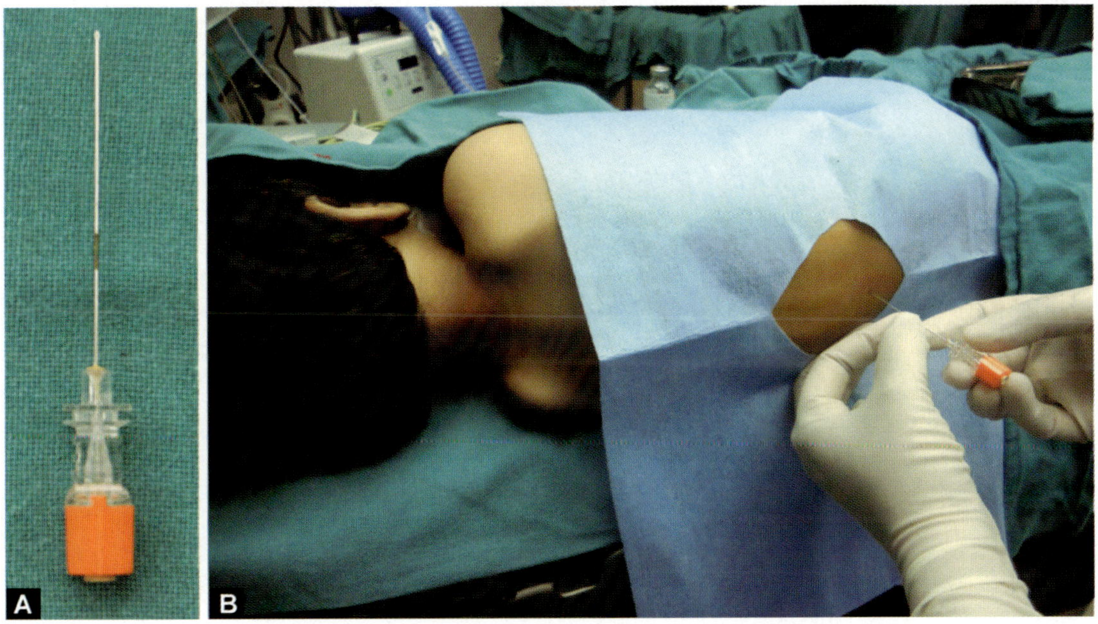

Figs 3.13A and B: (A) Spinal needle; (B) Spinal block

make them ideal for subarachnoid block in neonates and infants who have higher rates of CSF turnover and larger ratios of CSF volume to weight.

CLINICAL PEARLS FOR SAFETY AND EFFECTIVENESS OF SUBARACHNOID BLOCK

1. Monitoring of SpO_2 is essential to ensure patient safety.
2. Hypobaric solution/Barbotage method/Trendelenburg position/elevation of legs for placement of cautery pad are to be avoided to prevent unacceptably high level or total spinal block.
3. Timing of feeding is important as crying by hungry child makes surgery difficult. The child can be quietened with a pacifier or cotton ball soaked with 25% dextrose. Prolonged fasting may lead to hypotension following a sympathetic block.
4. In case of rapidly rising block, reverse Trendelenburg position is used.
5. Primarily limited to situations where general anesthesia/sedation poses excessive risk of apneic events and prolonged mechanical ventilation as in ex premature infants and neurologically impaired children.

Table 3.11: Dosage regime of local anesthetics for spinal block

Drug	*Dose (mg kg^{-1})*	*Vol (ml/kg)*	*Duration (min)*
• Bupivacaine 0.5%			
0-5 kg	0.5	0.1	65-75
5-15 kg	0.4	0.08	70-80
>15 kg	0.3	0.06	75-85
• Tetracaine 1%	0.5-1 (diluted with an equal volume of 10% dextrose with epinephrine 'wash')		

ADVERSE EFFECTS

Uncommon in children but may include hypotension, bradycardia, postdural puncture headache, transient radicular symptoms, intravascular injection or total spinal block with respiratory arrest and bradycardia.

COMBINED SPINAL EPIDURAL ANALGESIA

Combined spinal epidural analgesia (CSEA) is a potential option to GA for major abdominal surgery in infants.

CONTRAINDICATIONS FOR NEURAXIAL BLOCK

1. Parental refusal
2. Sepsis
3. Meningomyelocele
4. Hydrocephalus
5. Coagulopathy
6. Elevated intracranial pressure.

Infraorbital Nerve Block

ANATOMY

The infraorbital nerve is the termination of the second division of the trigeminal nerve. It is entirely sensory. It emerges in front of the maxilla through the infraorbital foramen and divides into branches to supply the lower eyelid, inferolateral part of the nose and upper lip with the mucosa **(Fig. 3.14A)**.

INDICATIONS

- Cleft-lip repair
- Nasal septum reconstruction
- Rhinoplasty
- Endoscopic sinus surgery
- Transsphenoidal hypophysectomy
- Facial trauma involving upper lip and inframaxillary area.

TECHNIQUES

Intraoral Approach (Fig. 3.14B)

After palpating the infraorbital foramen along the inferior rim of the orbit the upper lip is folded back. A 27G needle is inserted through the superior buccal groove and directed to the infraorbital foramen. After careful aspiration, 0.5 to 1 ml of 0.25% bupivacaine is injected.

Extraoral Approach (Fig. 3.14C)

After palpating the infraorbital notch the same volume is injected directly through the skin.

COMPLICATIONS

Swelling and ecchymoses of lower eyelid.

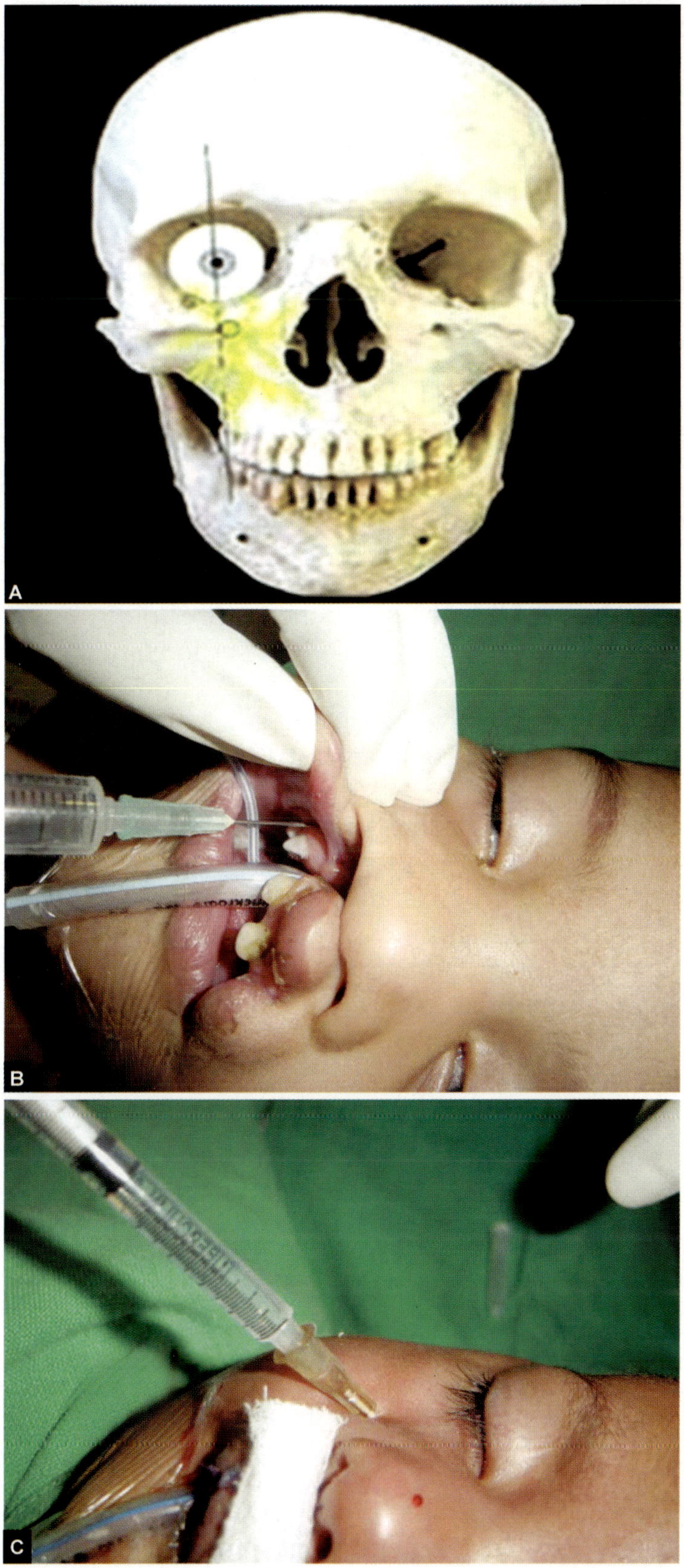

Figs 3.14A to C: (A) Anatomy of infraorbital nerve; (B) Intraoral approach; (C) Extraoral approach

Brachial Plexus Block

It can be performed through four approaches:
- Axillary
- Interscalene
- Supraclavicular
- Infraclavicular

AXILLARY APPROACH (FIGS 3.15A TO C)

It is the safest, most reliable and most commonly used site in neonates and children.

INDICATIONS

1. Upper extremity surgery
2. Sympathetic block following reimplantation surgery.

TECHNIQUE

1. Landmark and positioning are the same as in the adult. Supine position with arm abducted to 90 degrees and rotated externally with forearm flexed 90 degrees at elbow to make the plexus easily palpable.
2. A 22G short bevelled needle is inserted at 90 degrees to the skin just superior to the axillary artery pulsation at most proximal point against the upper part of humerus until a fascial click is felt.
3. After negative aspiration for blood, local anesthetic is injected. Distal tourniquet or digital massage helps proximal spread of drug.
4. Transarterial approach is not recommended.
5. Paresthesia is not required, so suitable in anesthetized patients.
6. Continuous plexus block through catheter technique can also be done.
7. Since the plexus is more superficial in children, too deep an injection is the common cause for failure.

DOSAGE

- Lidocaine 1–1.5% with epinephrine – 0.5 ml/kg, provides 3-4 hours of analgesia.
- Bupivacaine 0.25%—0.5 ml/kg, provides 8–10 hours of analgesia.

Intercostal Block

INDICATIONS

Thoracic and abdominal surgical procedures.

KEY ANATOMY (FIGS 3.16A AND B)

1. Intercostal vessels and nerves traverse the middle of the intercostal space posteriorly, where the local anesthesia is deposited. It is important to aspirate for blood to avoid intravascular injections.
2. At the paravertebral gutter the pleura and fascia are loosely attached to the ribs—allowing easy spread of local anesthetic to the adjacent intercostal spaces.

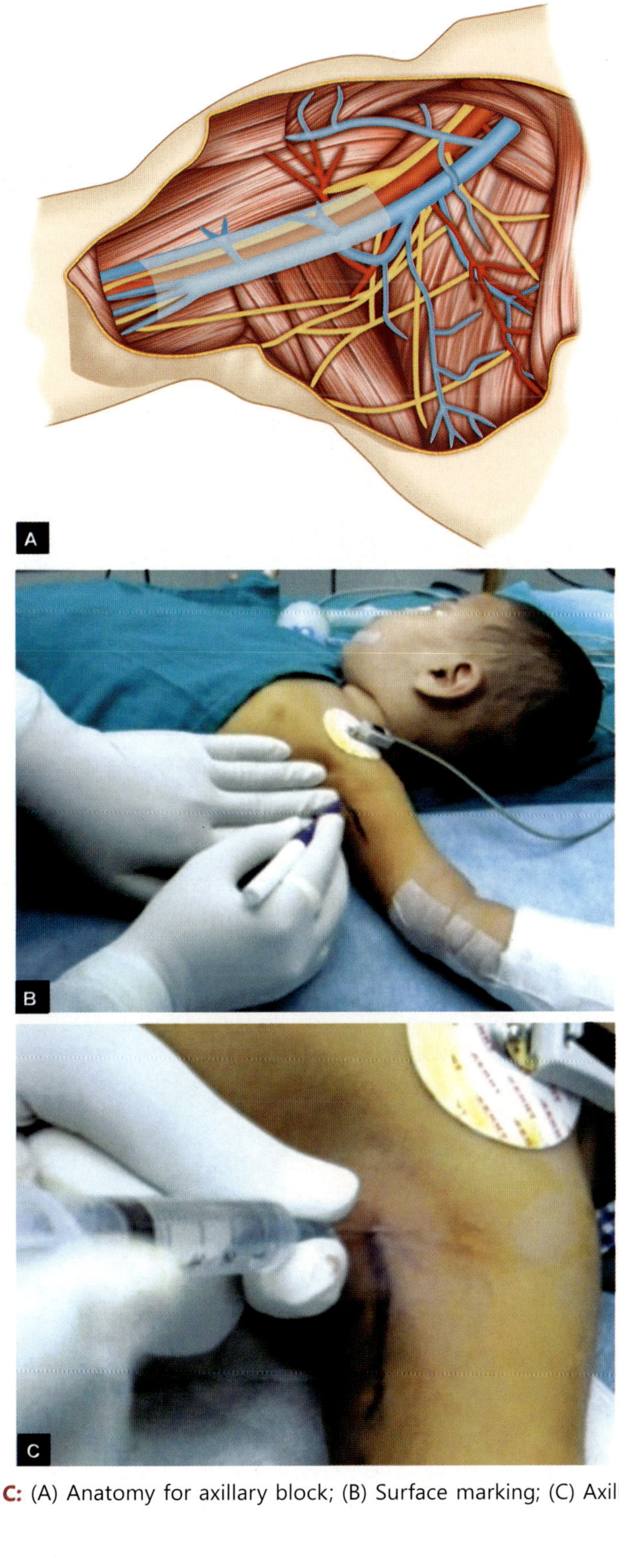

Figs 3.15A to C: (A) Anatomy for axillary block; (B) Surface marking; (C) Axillary nerve block

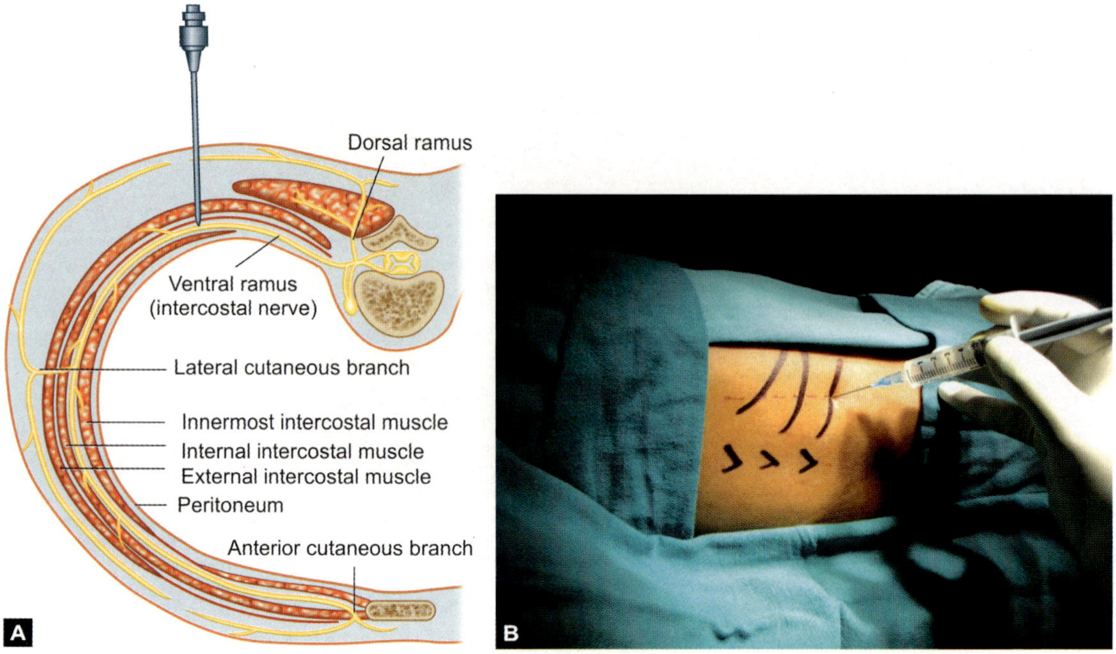

Figs 3.16A and B: (A) Anatomy for intercostal nerve block; (B) Intercostal nerve block

3. Bilateral block is better tolerated in infants as respiration in this age group is mainly diaphragmatic.

TECHNIQUE

The needle is inserted at right angles just lateral to paravertebral muscle onto the rib above and then walked down until it passes under the rib. A grating sensation is felt on piercing the posterior intercostal membrane and then into the intercostal space. Local anesthetic is injected after stabilizing the needle with the left hand to avoid injury to lung, pleura during coughing. Volume of local anesthetic depends upon the weight of the child and single or multiple injections. Since uptake is rapid, local anesthetic with epinephrine is preferred.

DOSAGE

0.3 ml/kg, 0.25% bupivacaine with adrenaline is required for each intercostal space.

Paravertebral Block (Figs 3.17A and B)

INDICATIONS

An alternative to epidural or intercostal block for thoracic procedures, renal surgery or cholecystectomy.

TECHNIQUE

With the patient in a lateral position, the tips of the vertebral spinous processes are marked at the target level. The distance from midline to the site of puncture is equal to the distance between two spinous processes.

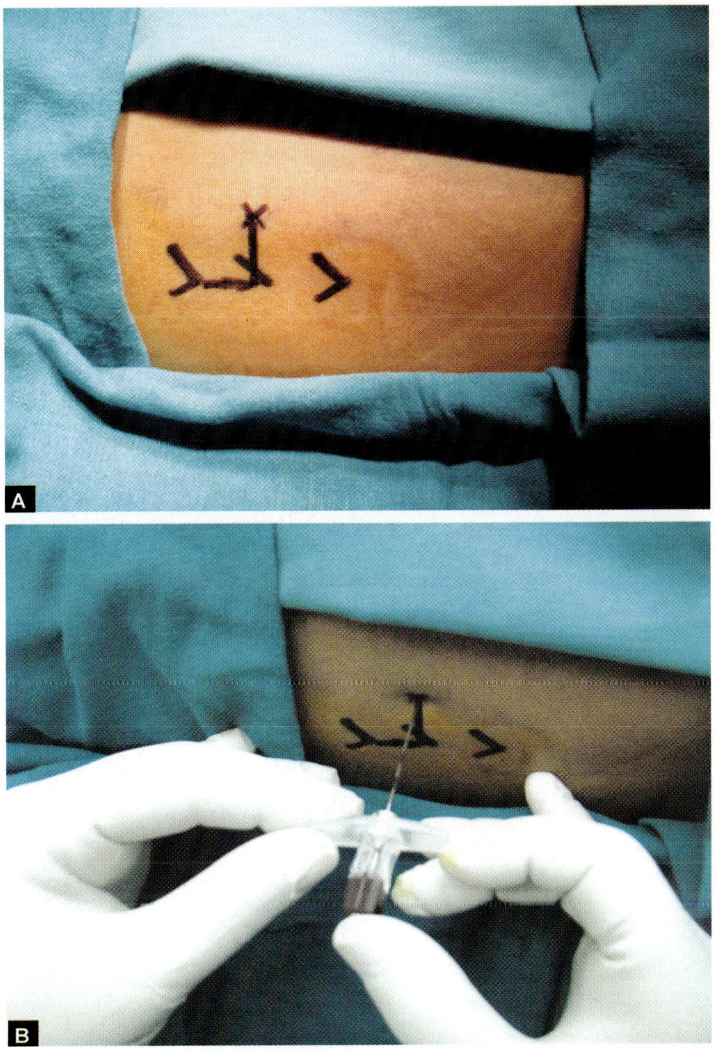

Figs 3.17A and B: (A) Surface marking for paravertebral block; (B) Paravertebral block

FORMULA

Distance (mm) = 0.12 x weight (kg) + 0.12
Depth (mm) = 0.48 x weight (kg) + 18.7

A small gauge Tuohy needle or spinal needle is inserted at right angle to the skin at the target site till the transverse process is contacted. Then the needle is attached to a saline-filled syringe and walked over to traverse the costotransverse ligament with loss of resistance technique.

DOSAGE

0.5 ml/kg, 0.25% bupivacaine at desired level (not more than 5 ml per level). Do not exceed maximum allowable dose with multiple injections. If a catheter technique is required, 0.25% bupivacaine with epinephrine 1:200,000 is infused at the rate of 0.25 ml/kg/hr.

COMPLICATIONS

Potential hazard of dural puncture in case of an extended dural cuff, vascular puncture.

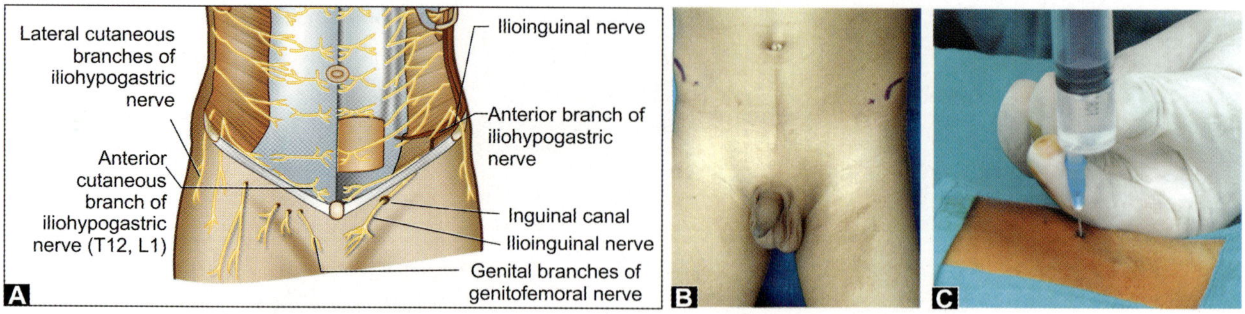

Figs 3.18A to C: (A) Anatomy for ILIH block; (B) Surface landmark; (C) ILIH block

Ilioinguinal and Iliohypogastric Nerve Block (ILIH) (Figs 3.18A to C)

INDICATIONS

Inguinal herniorrhaphy, orchidopexy.

ANATOMY

Both the nerves are derived from L_1 and eventually pierce the internal oblique muscle just below and medial to the anterior superior iliac spine to run between it and the external oblique (EO) aponeurosis. The hernia sac lies between the internal oblique (IO) and transversus abdominis (TA).

TECHNIQUE

A 22 G short bevel needle is inserted perpendicular to the skin 1-2 cm medial to the anterior superior iliac spine until a give is felt with penetration of the external oblique aponeurosis. After negative aspiration 0.25 ml/kg of 0.25% bupivacaine is injected. Then the needle is slowly advanced with pressure on the plunger to enter deep to the internal oblique. Again the same amount of local anesthetic is injected which can be massaged easily towards the neck of hernia sac. The block is repeated on the other side for bilateral inguinal herniotomy.

ADVANTAGE

Safe, effective for all ages.

DISADVANTAGES

Transient femoral nerve block, colonic perforation.

Transversus Abdominis Plane Block (TAP Block) (Figs 3.19A and B)

It is an abdominal field block.

INDICATIONS

Lower abdominal surgery (appendicectomy, hernia), laparoscopic surgery.

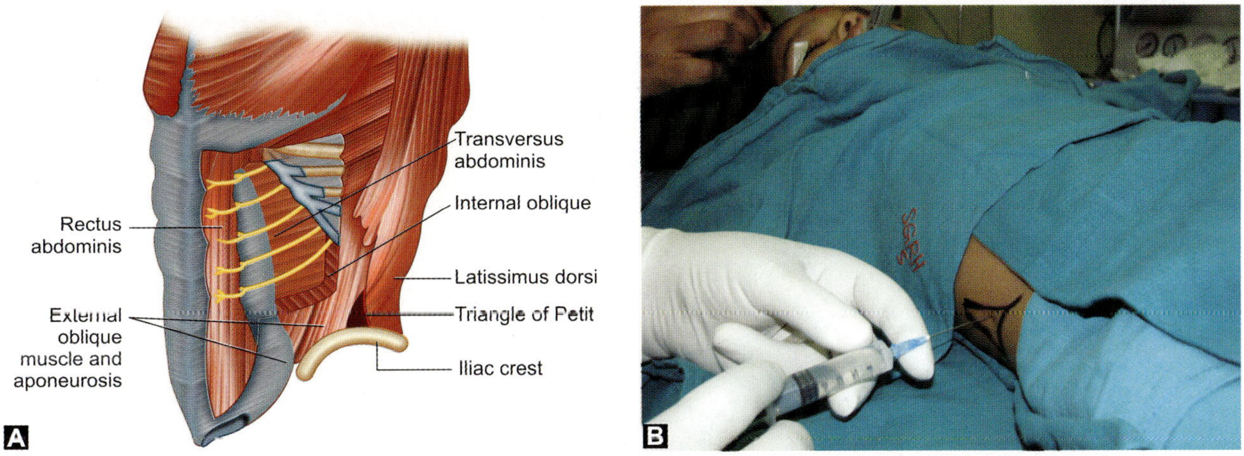

Figs 3.19A and B: (A) Anatomy of IAP block; (B) Surface marking and TAP block injection

ANATOMY

The anterior abdominal wall (skin, muscles and parietal peritoneum) is innervated by the anterior rami of lower thoracic (T_6-T_{12}) and first lumbar (iliohypogastric, ilioinguinal) nerves. The intermuscular plane between IO and TA muscles is called the transversus abdominis plane (TAP). There is a fascial sheath between internal oblique and transversus abdominis muscle. T_6-T_9 nerves enter the TAP medial to the anterior axillary line while T_{10}-L_1 nerves run in the TAP lateral to the anterior axillary line.

The terminal branches of these somatic nerves course through the lateral abdominal wall forming a TAP plexus due to extensive branching deep to the fascia and run with the deep circumflex iliac artery.

TECHNIQUE

The aim is to deposit local anesthetic in the TAP targeting these spinal nerves. The technique is landmark-guided, involving needle insertion at the lumbar triangle of Petit. This triangle lies above the pelvic brim in mid-axillary line bounded by latissimus dorsi posteriorly, EO muscle anteriorly and iliac crest inferiorly as the base of the triangle. It can be performed blind or by using ultrasound and single injection or continuous technique. Ultrasound guided TAP block promises better localization and deposition of LA with improved accuracy.

A 24G blunt-tipped 50 mm needle is inserted perpendicular to the skin just above the iliac crest and posterior to mid-axillary line within the triangle of Petit looking for a tactile end-point of double pops. The first pop indicates penetration of EO fascia and entry into the plane between EO and IO muscles, the second pop signifies penetration of fascial sheath in between IO and TA muscles and entry into TAP.

Following a single injection, unilateral good analgesia is expected in T_{10}-L_1 innervation. Augmentation with a subcostal injection attains a higher block up to T_7. For subcostal TAP, the needle is introduced from the lateral side of rectus muscle at the costal margin. For prolonged analgesia, a catheter is introduced into the TAP through a Tuohy needle. After opening up the plane with 2 ml saline the catheter is introduced approximately 3 cm beyond the needle tip.

DOSE

The volume of injectate is critical to the success of TAP block.

- Single injection of 20 ml of diluted solution of bupivacaine/ropivacaine on each side (maximum recommended dose should not be exceeded).
- For smaller children 0.5-1 ml/kg of 0.25% bupivacaine may be considered.
- Catheter technique:
  - Infusion of 7-10 ml/hr of diluted LA following 20 ml bolus.
  - Bilateral injection for midline incision
  - Subcostal TAP –10 ml of LA extends block above umbilicus.

COMPLICATIONS

- Intraperitoneal injection
- Hematoma
- Bowel perforation
- Transient femoral nerve palsy
- Intrahepatic injection.

Penile Block (Figs 3.20A to C)

INDICATIONS

Circumcision, distal hypospadias repair, meatotomy.

ANATOMY

The principal innervation of the penis is via two dorsal penile nerves (S_2, S_3, S_4).

Each dorsal nerve emerges under the symphysis pubis and runs down the shaft of the penis beneath the Buck's fascia. The nerves lie in a triangular compartment in the subpubic space; bounded by the symphysis pubis above, corpora cavernosa below and the membranous layer of fascia in front. The fascia splits in its deep surface to form the vertical suspensory ligament of the penis which in turn divides to encircle the shaft of the penis.

Thus, the subpubic space is divided into two potential spaces on either side of the suspensory ligament which usually do not communicate directly.

The dorsal nerves and vessels lie deep to the suspensory ligament in an enclosed triangle where they can be compressed if a large hematoma develops.

TECHNIQUE

The pubic symphysis is the anatomical landmark. The penis is pulled down to open the subpubic space and a 23 – 25G, 3 cm long needle with a short bevel is inserted at right angle to the skin in the midline until it touches the symphysis pubis as a guide to depth. The needle is withdrawn slightly and then redirected to pass below the symphysis pubis at 15° to the midline into the potential space marked by a 'pop'—penetration of the fascia. After negative aspiration the calculated local anesthetic is injected. Then the needle is withdrawn up to the subcutaneous tissue and reinserted on the other side at a 15° angle to deposit an equal volume of local anesthetic.

DOSAGE

0.5% bupivacaine (1 ml + 0.1 ml/kg) for each side is recommended.

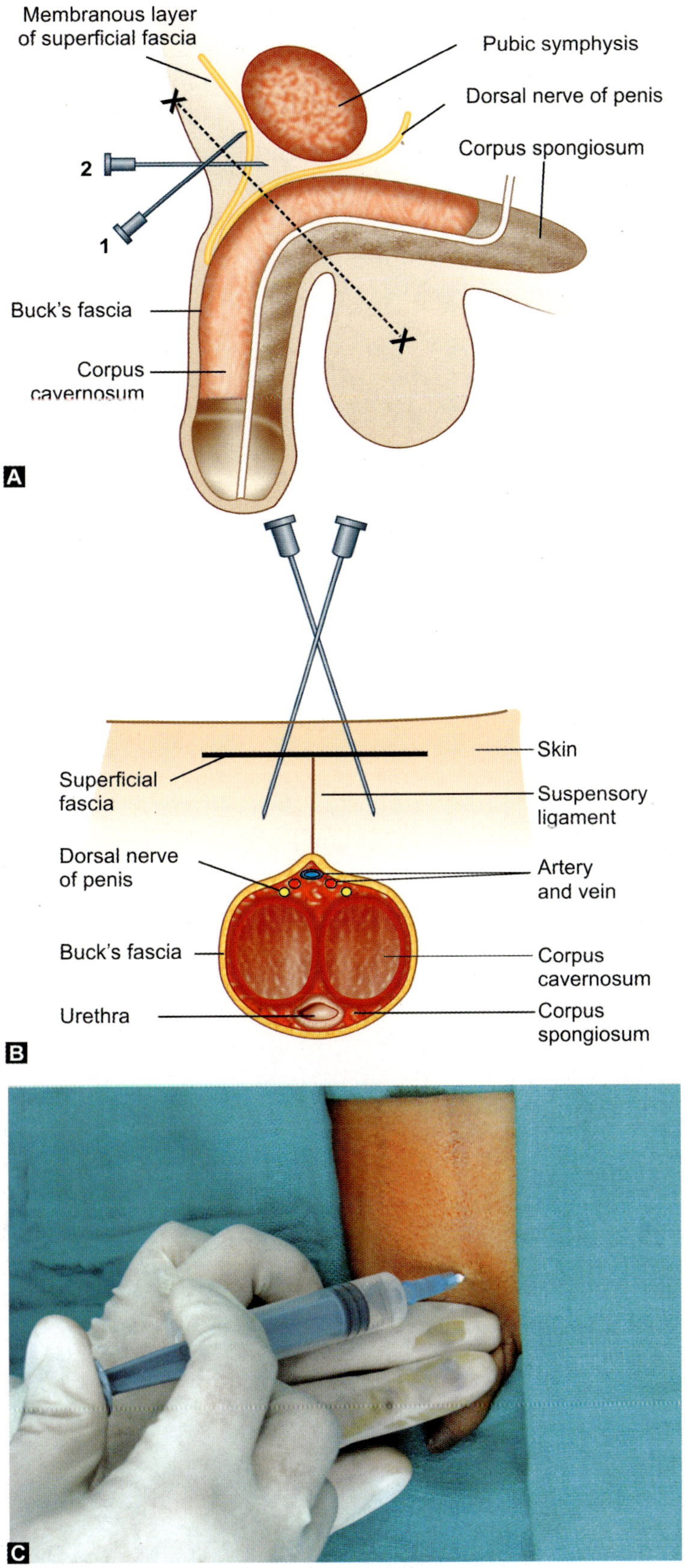

Figs 3.20A to C: Penile anatomy (A) Sagittal plane; (B) Coronal plane; (C) Penile block

KEY POINTS FOR A SAFE AND EFFECTIVE BLOCK

1. Avoid midline injection to reduce injury to dorsal vessels and subsequent hematoma.
2. Always aspirate before injecting to ensure that the needle has not penetrated a blood vessel or the corpus cavernosum.
3 Epinephrine is absolutely contraindicated as it can lead to the spasm of the dorsal artery with subsequent ischemia and necrosis of the glans.
4 Adequate volume of local anesthetic is required so that the solution can pass posteriorly to block the ventral branch supplying the frenulum.

OTHER METHODS

1. *Lateral approach/Two injection technique:* After gently pulling the penis downwards, two injections are made perpendicular to the skin just below each of the pubic rami at 10.30 o' clock and 1.30 o' clock position just beneath the Buck's fascia. The fascia is approximately 3–5 mm below the skin surface.
2. *Subcutaneous ring block:* It is technically easy and very effective. 0.25-0.5% bupivacaine (1-5 ml) is infiltrated circumferentially superficial to Buck's fascia around the base of penis forming a visible wheal.

Femoral Nerve Block (Figs 3.21A and B)

INDICATIONS

Fracture shaft of femur, skin graft from thigh, quadriceps muscle biopsy and transportation of children with fracture femur for X-ray, etc.

ANATOMY

The femoral nerve lies just lateral to the femoral artery below the inguinal ligament deep to the fascia lata and fascia iliaca.

TECHNIQUE

In the supine position with feet rotated outward, a 5 cm, 22 G short bevelled needle is inserted at a 45° angle to the skin just 0.5-1 cm lateral to the artery and 0.5-1 cm below the inguinal ligament. The needle is directed cephalad and slightly medially towards the umbilicus till loss of resistance is felt twice. If injection of local anesthetic is smooth, the needle is in the femoral canal. If there is a resistance to injection, the needle is withdrawn and advanced again with gentle pressure on the plunger till injection becomes smooth.

DOSAGE

0.3–0.5 ml/kg of 0.2% ropivacaine or 0.25% bupivacaine. The volume is doubled for a 3-in-1 block to spread adequately between fascia iliaca and muscle to reach the lateral cutaneous nerve of the thigh and the obturator nerve. Employing distal pressure during injection may result in cephalad spread.

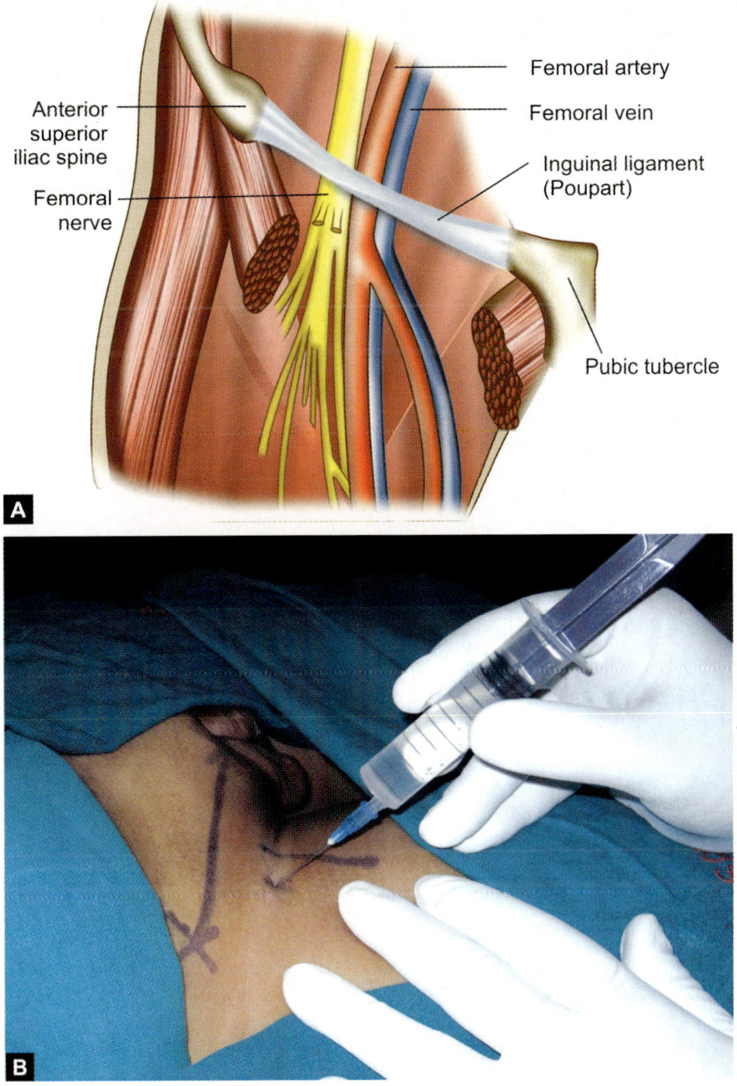

Figs 3.21A and B: (A) Anatomy of femoral nerve block; (B) Surface marking and femoral block

Psoas Compartment Block (PCB) (Figs 3.22A and B)

INDICATIONS

Surgery of hip, femoral shaft or knee.

ANATOMY

The term 'psoas compartment block' was coined by Chayen and colleagues to describe loss of resistance technique for the injection of local anesthetic into the 'compartment' between the quadratus lumborum posteriorly and psoas major inferiorly. It consistently blocks the main components of the lumbar plexus, namely the femoral nerve, lateral femoral cutaneous nerve and the obturator nerve as they run within the psoas major muscle.

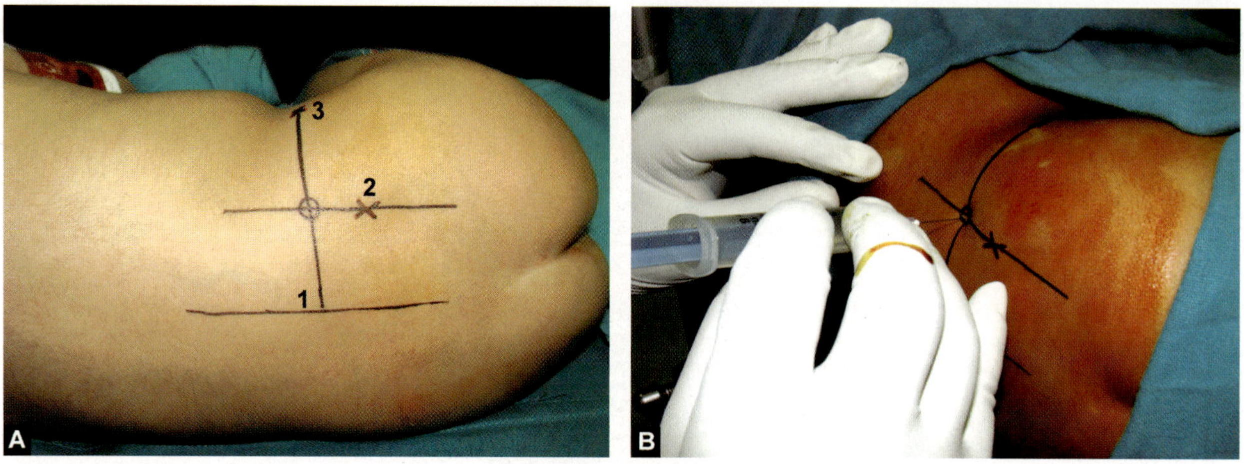

Figs 3.22A and B: (A) Surface marking for Psoas compartment block (1) spine, (2) PSIS, (3) Iliac crest; (B) PCB block

TECHNIQUE

The patient is placed in lateral decubitus position with the operative side uppermost. Two lines are drawn, i.e. one line is drawn joining the highest point of iliac crests and the other line is drawn parallel to the spinal column passing through the posterosuperior iliac spine (PSIS) of the superior side. The needle is inserted at 90 degrees to the skin at the intersection of these two lines and will traverse through the quadratus lumborum.

Ideally a nerve stimulator is recommended with elicitation of response to stimulation of foot. Careful aspiration before injection and fractionation of injectate is important.

ADVANTAGES

It is an alternative to epidural analgesia in hip procedures where access to the epidural space is difficult.

Continuous infusion analgesia is possible.

It obviates the use of bilateral blockade in unilateral surgery.

If combined with sciatic nerve block, it provides anesthesia for whole lower limb unilaterally.

COMPLICATIONS

- Intravenous injection and systemic toxicity
- Total spinal block
- Retroperitoneal injection.

Fascia Iliaca Compartment Block (Figs 3.23A and B)

- Provides very good analgesia for surgical procedures involving the thigh, knee and mid-leg.
- Provides anesthesia of femoral nerve (100%), lateral femoral cutaneous (90%) and obturator (75%) nerves by a spread of anesthetic behind fascia iliaca.

TECHNIQUE

A short bevel needle is inserted perpendicular to the skin 0.5–1 cm below the junction of lateral one-third and medial two-third of inguinal ligament. Two "pops" should be felt as both fascia lata and fascia iliaca are pierced. Then after negative aspiration for blood, local anesthetic is

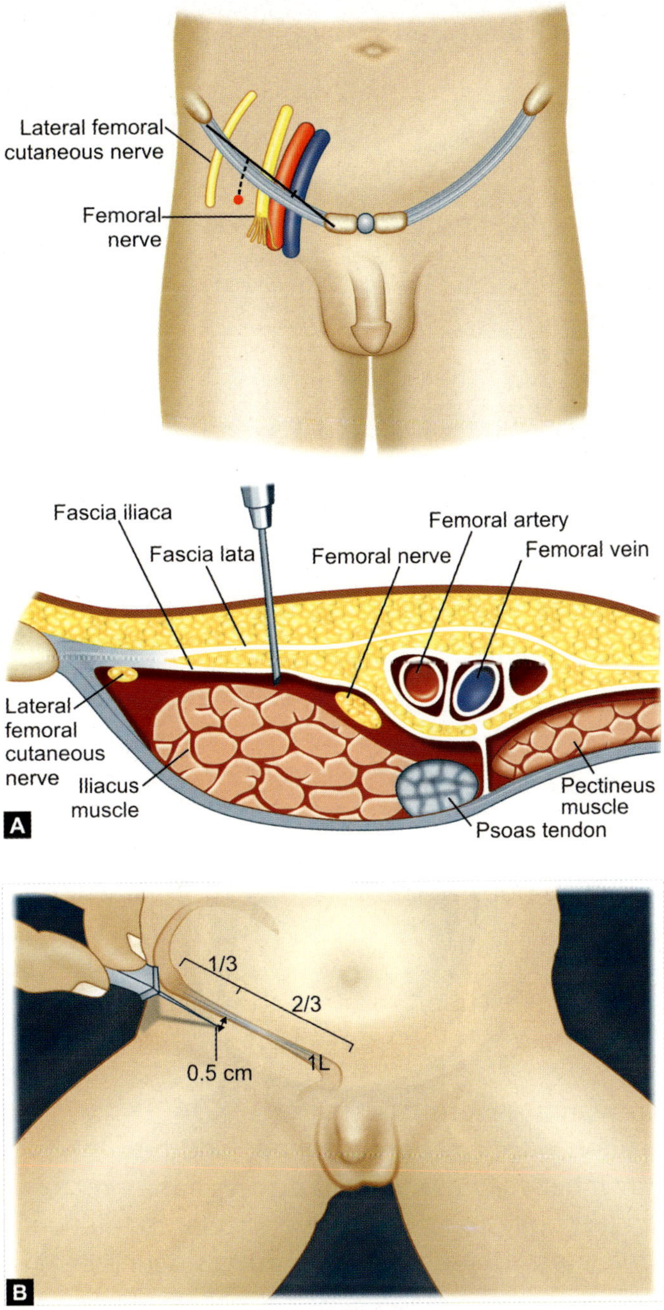

Figs 3.23A and B: (A) Anatomy for fascia iliaca block; (B) Fascia iliaca compartment block

injected slowly without any resistance or visible skin wheal and with distal digital pressure to facilitate cephalad spread.

DOSE

0.5 ml/kg of 0.2% ropivacaine or 0.25% bupivacaine.

COMPLICATION

Femoral artery puncture—apply pressure for 5 minutes to prevent a hematoma.

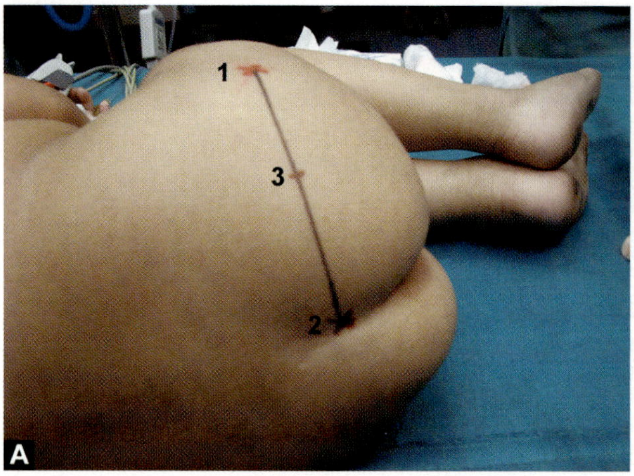

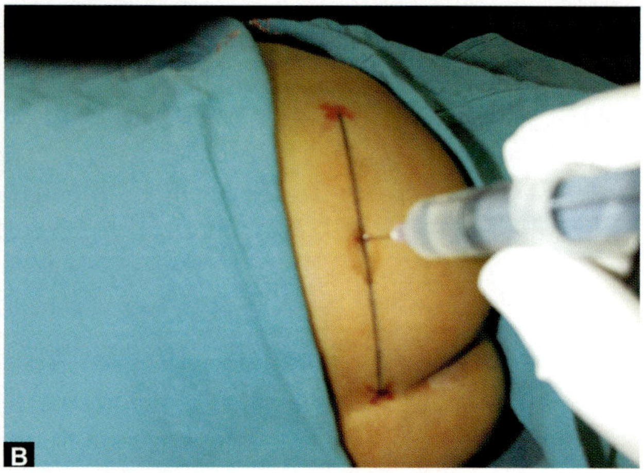

Figs 3.24A and B: (A) Surface marking for sciatic nerve block: (1) Greater trochanter (2) tip of coccyx (3) injection site; (B) Sciatic nerve block

Sciatic Nerve Block (Figs 3.24A and B)

Sciatic nerve is derived from L_4-S_3.

INDICATIONS

Distal lower extremity procedures.

DRUG

0.5–1 ml/kg of 0.25% or 0.5 % bupivacaine.

TECHNIQUE

Several approaches have been described to block the sciatic nerve.

POSTERIOR APPROACH

Easier and more reliable than anterior or lateral approach:
- Lateral decubitus position with legs flexed at knee and hip.
- An imaginary line drawn between the tip of the coccyx and greater trochanter of femur. The needle is inserted at mid-point of this line, perpendicular to the skin, then advanced medially and upward toward the lateral border of ischial tuberosity until a muscle twitch is seen in the foot.

Popliteal Fossa Block (Figs 3.25A and B)

In the prone or supine position the leg is lifted with knee and thigh flexed. The sciatic nerve emerges into the popliteal fossa near the superior apex of the diamond shaped area formed by the (biceps femoris—laterally, semitendinosus and semimembranosus—medially and inferiorly by the two heads of gastrocnemius). With the help of a nerve stimulator, a needle is inserted just caudad and lateral to the superior apex of the fossa lateral to the popliteal artery- while the foot is observed for plantar or dorsiflexion.

DOSE

Larger volume of local anesthetic (0.75–1 ml/kg) of 0.25-0.5% bupivacaine is required.

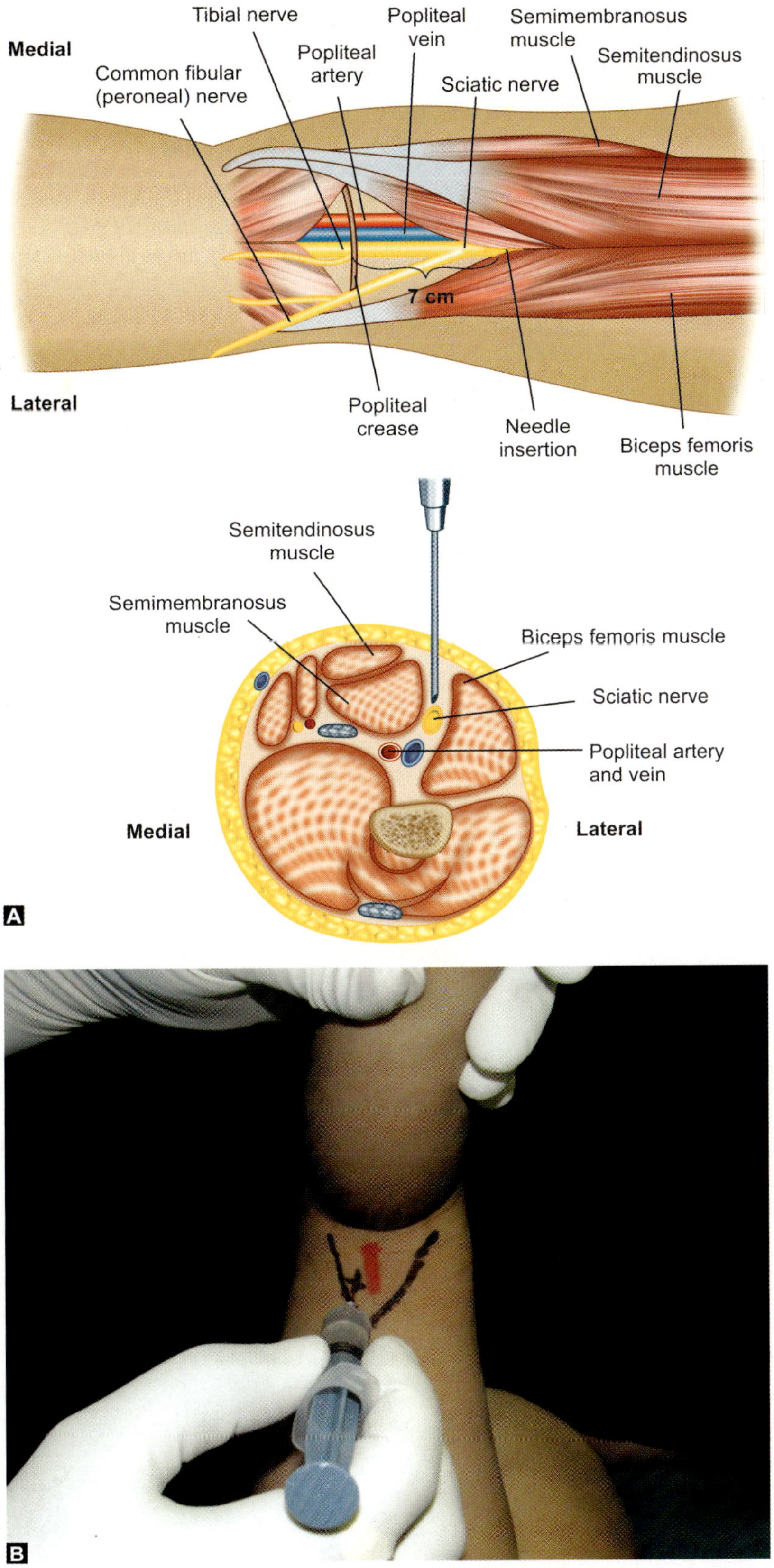

Figs 3.25A and B: Popliteal fossa block

4 Procedural Sedation and Analgesia

Sedation and analgesia in pediatric patients for diagnostic and therapeutic procedures outside the operating room is becoming more frequent as health care is being driven to be efficient and cost-effective.

Objective

The goal is to minimize discomfort, pain or any negative psychological response while making it possible to do the procedure properly and on completion, the patient should return to the pre-procedural state for safe discharge.

Levels of Sedation

The JCAHO (Joint Commission for Accreditation of Health Organization) defines four levels of sedation and anesthesia on recommendations made by the ASA (American Society of Anesthesiologists) for anesthesiologists and non-anesthesiologists with a strong emphasis on safety **(Table 4.1)**.

MINIMAL SEDATION (ANXIOLYSIS)

It is a drug induced state that allows a normal response to verbal commands. Though cognitive and motor function may be impaired, but airway, ventilation and cardiovascular function remain unaffected.

Table 4.1: Levels of sedation

	Minimal sedation/ Anxiolysis	*Moderate sedation/ analgesia*	*Deep sedation*	*General anesthesia*
Responsiveness	Normal response to verbal stimulation	Purposeful response to verbal commands or light touch	Purposeful response to verbal, repeated tactile or painful stimulation	Unarousable even to repeated or painful stimulation
Airway	Unaffected	No intervention required	Intervention may be required	Intervention often required
Spontaneous ventilation	Unaffected	Adequate	May be inadequate	Frequently inadequate
Cardiovascular function	Unaffected	Usually maintained	Usually maintained	May be impaired

MODERATE SEDATION/ANALGESIA (CONSCIOUS SEDATION)

A drug induced depression of consciousness during which patients respond purposefully to verbal commands either alone or accompanied by light tactile stimulation. The airway remains patent without intervention, adequate spontaneous ventilation and cardiovascular function are usually maintained. The old terminology of "conscious sedation" is no longer used.

DEEP SEDATION/ANALGESIA

A drug induced depression of consciousness during which patients cannot be easily aroused but respond purposefully following repeated or painful stimulation. Cardiovascular function is usually maintained, but may require assistance to maintain airway and ventilation.

GENERAL ANESTHESIA

A drug induced loss of consciousness during which patients are not arousable, even by painful stimulation. They often require assistance in maintaining a patent airway and ventilation. Cardiovascular function may be impaired.

Levels of sedation are not discrete. Sedation is continuum and it is not possible to draw clear cut lines between various levels of sedation. There is always potential for losing protective airway reflexes once a child crosses the threshold of deep sedation **(Fig. 4.1)**.

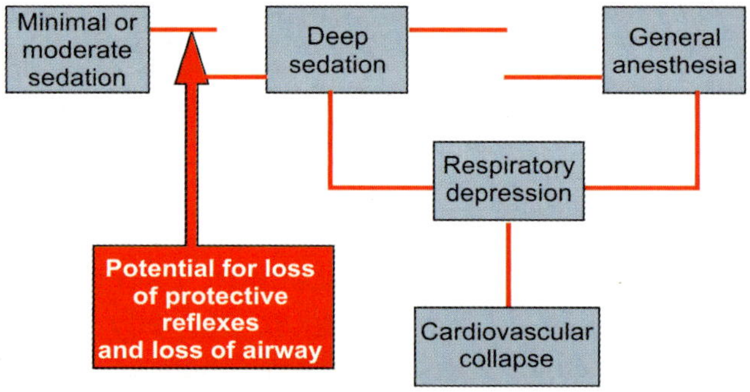

Fig. 4.1: Sedation continuum

Preparation for Sedation

PRE-SEDATION ASSESSMENT

- Medical history
- Airway assessment
- NPO status—strictly followed as for general anesthesia **(Fig. 4.2)**
- Weight record
- Laboratory investigations as required.

NPO Guidelines	
Solids/Milk formula	6 hours
Breast milk	3-4 hours
Clear liquid	2 hours

Fig. 4.2: Fasting policy

DOCUMENTATION

- Informed consent of parents or relatives
- Standardized sedation record to be maintained, which also includes baseline vital signs and trends during sedation period.

CHOICE OF DRUGS (TABLE 4.2)

Depends upon:
- Type of procedure
- Duration of procedure
- Need of amnesia

Table 4.2: Commonly used drugs for sedation and analgesia			
Name	*Dosage*	*Route*	*Clinical Significance*
Midazolam	0.5–0.75 mg kg^{-1} 0.02–0.20 mg kg^{-1} 0.25 mg kg^{-1}	Oral IV Nasal	Nasal route – irritating
Chloral hydrate	50-100 mg kg^{-1}	Oral	Used for painless radio-diagnostic procedure Prolonged sedation Paradoxical agitation
Propofol	Bolus 1 mg kg^{-1} followed by 0.25-0.5 mg kg^{-1} bolus every 1-2 minutes	IV	Pain on injection Useful for non-painful procedures Transient apnea and hypotension
	100-200 mcg kg^{-1} min^{-1}	IV infusion	
Ketamine	2-3 mg kg^{-1} 0.5-1 mg kg^{-1} 6-8 mg kg^{-1}	IM IV PO/PR	Useful in painful procedure Dissociative anesthesia Nausea, vomiting, Hallucination, emergence-delirium prevented by midazolam and fentanyl Laryngospasm – anticholinergic given to minimize secretions Contraindicated in active respiratory infection, seizure disorders
Remifentanil	0.1 mcg kg^{-1} min^{-1}	IV infusion	Apnea is a significant risk Short half-life
N_2O	50 : 50 in O_2	Inhalation	For moderately painful procedure
Dexmedetomidine	1 mcg kg^{-1} bolus 0.5-0.7 mcg kg^{-1} hr^{-1}	IV IV infusion	For cardiac catheterization, awake craniotomies, burns dressing
Midazolam + Fentanyl	Midazolam 0.02 mg kg^{-1} Fentanyl 1-2 mcg kg^{-1}	IV IV	Most common combination in use
Propofol + Fentanyl	Propofol 50-100 mcg kg^{-1} Fentanyl 1-2 mcg kg^{-1}	IV IV	For deep sedation Requires airway management

- Requirement of immobility
- Need of loss of consciousness
- Posture and position during procedure.

The pharmacological actions required are sedation, hypnosis, analgesia, amnesia and akinesia. The commonly used drugs can be categorized as:

- *Mainly sedatives* → barbiturates, chloral hydrate, benzodiazepines, propofol
- *Mainly analgesics* → acetaminophen, NSAIDs, opioids, local anesthetics
- *Both sedative-analgesics* → ketamine, nitrous oxide.

Clinical Pearls for Procedural Sedation

- Sleep deprivation before sedation should be encouraged
- Elective sedation should be avoided in case of optimizable problems such as fever, significant cough, sputum production
- Titrate the minimum effective dose to achieve desired level of sedation and analgesia.

Recommended Guidelines for Safe Sedation

- The sedation room should be fully equipped for resuscitation with:
  - Age appropriate equipment
  - Positive pressure O_2 delivery system
  - Suction apparatus and catheter
  - Standard resuscitation trolley
  - Emergency call system to summon additional help
  - In-facility for observation until fit for discharge
- Venous access must be secured and maintained
- Minimum monitoring
  - ECG
  - Blood pressure
  - Pulse oximetry
- Supplemental oxygen should be given to all patients
- During the procedure, any concern of adequacy of airway, ventilation or hemodynamic status should be addressed immediately, any other issue becomes second priority.

Recommended Discharge Criteria

- Post-sedation "Aldrete Score" should be 8-10
- Pre-sedation consciousness level should be achieved
- Patient should be able to speak, sit or walk (if age-appropriate)
- Respiratory and cardiovascular parameters should be stable and satisfactory
- Hydration should be adequate
- Pain should be easily controlled with oral analgesics
- A responsible adult should accompany the child on discharge
- The 'Helpline' contact number should be given to the escort in case of any need.

5 Pediatric Cardiopulmonary Resuscitation

The majority of cardiac arrests in infants and children are the terminal result of progressive respiratory failure or shock. This secondary cardiopulmonary arrest is also known as asphyxial arrest. The less frequent primary cardiac arrest caused by cardiac arrhythmias such as ventricular fibrillation (VF) or pulseless ventricular tachycardia (VT) is seen in approximately 5-15% of pediatric in-hospital and out of hospital cardiac arrests. These shockable rhythms are also seen in 27% of pediatric in-hospital arrest at some point during resuscitation. The incidence of VF and pulseless VT induced cardiac arrest rises with age.

Critical illness in children initially causes a variable period of systemic hypoxemia, hypercapnia and acidosis, progresses to bradycardia and hypotension and culminates in cardiac arrest. Since the outcome from cardiopulmonary resuscitation in children is poor, identification of the antecedent stages of cardiac or respiratory failure is a priority and effective early intervention may be life-saving. The goal of resuscitation is to urgently re-establish substrate delivery to meet the metabolic demands of vital organs by several specific interventions which form the pediatric basic life support (PBLS) and pediatric advanced life support (PALS).

Five distinct phases of cardiac arrest have been described:

1. Pre-arrest phase – requires early recognition and treatment of precipitating conditions and monitoring of high-risk children.
2. No-flow (cardiac arrest) phase – should be minimized as interval to BLS determines survival.
3. Low-flow cardiopulmonary resuscitation (CPR) phase—where the focus is on good quality CPR to produce optimal coronary perfusion.
4. Post-resuscitation phase (immediate) – concentrates on salvage of injured cells by providing them oxygen and achieving long-term survival.
5. Post-resuscitation phase (rehabilitation) focuses on early intervention with occupational and physical therapy.

In 2010, on the occasion of the 50th anniversary of the introduction of CPR, the American Heart Association (AHA) updated the existing guidelines for neonatal, pediatric and adult BLS and ALS protocols. Survival from in-hospital cardiac arrests in infants and children has changed favorably from 9% in 1980 to 17% in 2000 to 27% in 2006 whereas the overall survival to discharge from out-of-hospital cardiac arrest remains at 6% for last 20 years. Earlier recognition and management of at-risk in-patients by a formal pediatric medical emergency team (MET) or a rapid response team (RRT) and implementation of evidence based resuscitation guidelines may have played a role for this substantial improvement in outcome of in-hospital arrests. Infants have a higher survival rate than children whose survival rate is better than adults in in-hospital arrest.

Fig. 5.1: Pediatric chain of survival

AHA pediatric chain of survival comprises of 5 links, i.e. prevention, early CPR, prompt access to Emergency Response System (ERS), rapid PALS and integrated post-cardiac arrest care **(Fig. 5.1)**. The first 3 links of this chain constitute pediatric BLS.

Prevention of Cardiopulmonary Arrest

Causes of cardiac arrest in pediatric age group can be heterogeneous. In infants, the leading causes of death are congenital malformation, complications of prematurity and sudden infant death syndrome (SIDS). In children over 1 year of age, injury is the leading cause of death and survival from traumatic cardiac arrest is poor. Therefore, prevention of injury is very essential in reducing death and targeted interventions are emphasized to prevent motor vehicle accidents which are the most common cause of fatal childhood injuries.

Early BLS is significant and should be part of a community effort. Prompt and effective bystander CPR can be associated with successful return of spontaneous circulation (ROSC) with good neurologic outcome in out-of hospital cardiac arrest in children (> 70% survival in asphyxial arrest and 20-30% survival in sudden primary arrest). However, only about 30-50% of infants and children who suffer out-of-hospital cardiac arrest receive bystander CPR. Infants are less likely to survive out-of-hospital cardiac arrest most common cause being (SIDS) than children or adolescents. Survival is greater in initial rhythm of VF or pulseless VT than in those with asystole or pulseless electrical activity (PEA).

BLS Sequence

The 2010 AHA Guidelines for CPR recommend a CAB sequence (chest compressions, airway, breathing/ventilation) instead of ABC.

RATIONALE FOR THIS CHANGE

- The majority of victims requiring CPR are adults with VF cardiac arrest in whom early compression with minimal interruption is more important than ventilation for a better outcome. So beginning CPR with 30 compressions rather than 2 rescue breaths causes a shorter interval to first compression.
- Chest compression can be initiated immediately by all rescuers whereas ventilation (mouth-to-mouth or bag-mask ventilation) needs head positioning and attaining a seal which takes time and eventually delays the first compression.
- Chest compressions are crucial for keeping the blood circulating whereas there is a reserve of oxygen left in the patient's lungs and blood from the last breath.

In pediatric resuscitation, ventilations are extremely important because secondary cardio-pulmonary arrest is more common than primary VF cardiac arrest. CAB sequence theoretically

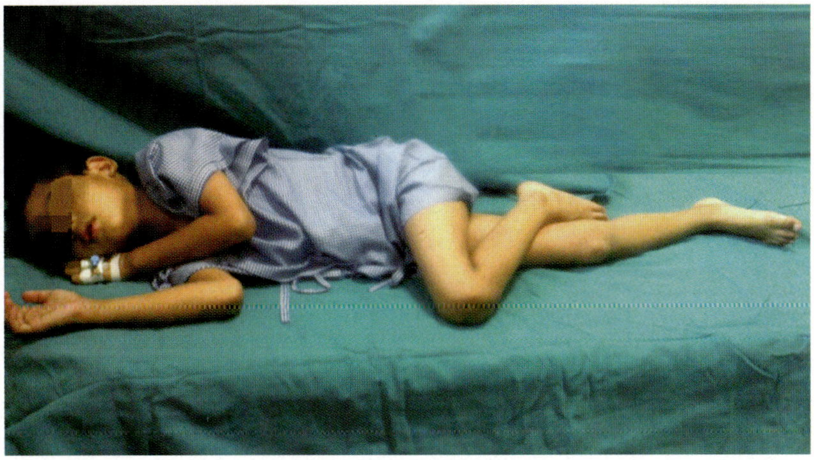

Fig. 5.2: Recovery position

delays ventilation by approximately 18 seconds for lone rescuer and even a shorter interval for 2 rescuers. However, CAB sequence is recommended in pediatric CPR to simplify training to rescuers with the hope that more victims of sudden cardiac arrest will receive bystander CPR.

- Infant BLS guidelines – for infants <1 year of age
- Child BLS guidelines – for 1 year of age until puberty
- Adult BLS guidelines – for children at and beyond puberty.

MANEUVERS RELATED TO CPR

Recovery Position

If the unresponsive child is breathing normally with a clear airway with no evidence of trauma, turn the child on his side in recovery position. An ideal recovery position helps maintain a patent airway with cervical spine stability, minimizes the risk of aspiration, limits pressure on bony prominences and peripheral nerves, enables the rescuer to observe the victim's respiratory effort and provides access to the victim for interventions **(Fig. 5.2)**.

Infants and small children should be turned on their side in a logroll manner so that head, shoulders and torso move as a single unit.

For older children, the following steps should be followed:

- Position yourself on the side of the victim.
- Place the arm nearest to you at right angle to the victim's body, elbow bent and palm up.
- Place the other arm across the chest so that the back of hand touches the cheek of the victim.
- Grasp the victim's far side thigh with right hand above the knee and flex it towards the body. Next hold the far side shoulder with left hand and roll the victim towards you onto his side.
- Adjust the upper leg so that the hip and knee are bent at right angles and lower leg is straight.
- Tilt the head back to open the airway using the upper hand under the cheek to maintain head tilt.

HIGH-QUALITY CHEST COMPRESSIONS

During cardiac arrest, high quality chest compressions generate blood flow to vital organs and increase the likelihood of ROSC. Cardiac compressions promote circulation of blood by direct compression of the heart between sternum and spine (cardiac pump), by increasing the thoracic pressure (thoracic pump) and by forcing blood from abdominal vessels to the periphery (abdominal pump). Out of these, the cardiac pump mechanism predominates in children as they have a compliant chest wall **(Fig. 5.3)**.

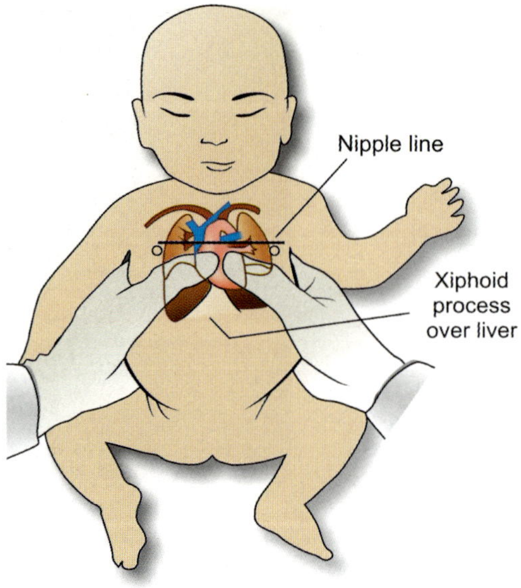

Fig. 5.3: Cardiac pump mechanism

- Push fast – at least 100 compressions per minute
- Push hard – depress to at least one-third of antero-posterior diameter of chest, i.e. 1.5 inch (4 cm) for infants, 2 inch (5 cm) for children
- Allow complete chest recoil after each compression to allow cardiac filling
- Minimize interruptions in compressions (except for ventilation until advanced airway in place, rhythm check, shock delivery) as every interruption stops blood flow to the brain which may lead to brain death if prolonged. Coronary perfusion pressure declines precipitously with interruption of chest compression. Thus, frequent interruptions in chest compressions may prolong the duration of low coronary perfusion pressure and flow which reduces the likelihood of ROSC. It takes several chest compressions to get the blood moving again to restore coronary and cerebral perfusion.
- Best results obtained if victim is lying on a firm surface.

Technique

Child

Compress the lower half of the sternum with the heel of one or both hands by lifting the fingers (do not compress xiphisternum or ribs). Position yourself vertically above the victim's chest and with your arms straight. In larger children or small rescuers, compression is most easily achieved by using both hands with the fingers interlocked **(Figs 5.4A and B)**.

Infant

- Two-finger technique for lone rescuer **(Fig. 5.5A)**
  Compress the sternum with tip of the two fingers placed just below the intermammary line (avoid compression over ribs or xiphoid process)

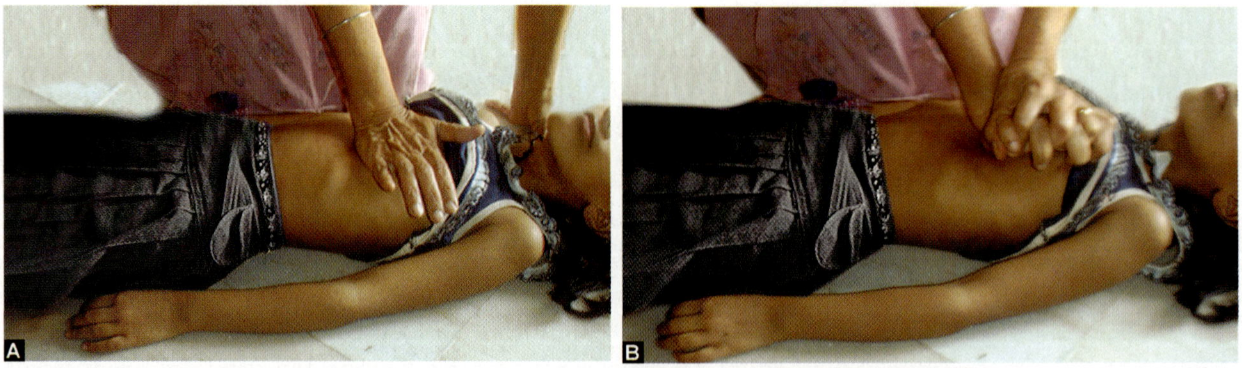

Figs 5.4A and B: (A) One hand method; (B) Two hand method

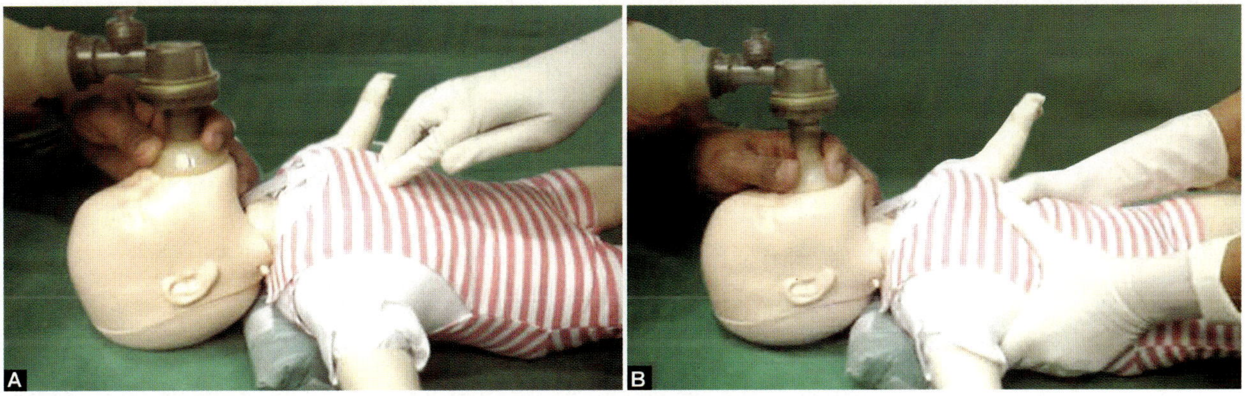

Figs 5.5A and B: (A) Two finger method; (B) Two thumb encircling hand method

- Two-thumb-encircling hand technique for two rescuers in case of health care providers (HCP) **(Fig. 5.5B)**

  Encircle the infant's chest with both hands, spread your fingers around the thorax and place your thumbs together over the lower half of sternum with the tips pointing towards infant's head. Compress the sternum forcefully with thumbs since a circumferential squeeze of the thorax shows doubtful benefit. However, this technique is preferred to the former as it produces higher coronary perfusion pressure, systolic and diastolic pressures and generates high-quality compression in relation to depth or force of compression.

Rescuer fatigue deteriorates compression quality (rate, depth, recoil), therefore rotate the compressor role every 2 minutes (>1 rescuer) and the switch should be accomplished as quickly as possible (<5 seconds) to minimize interruptions in chest compression.

OPEN AIRWAY AND GIVE VENTILATION (FIG. 5.6)

Child

Open the airway by head tilt and chin lift (without overextension of neck).

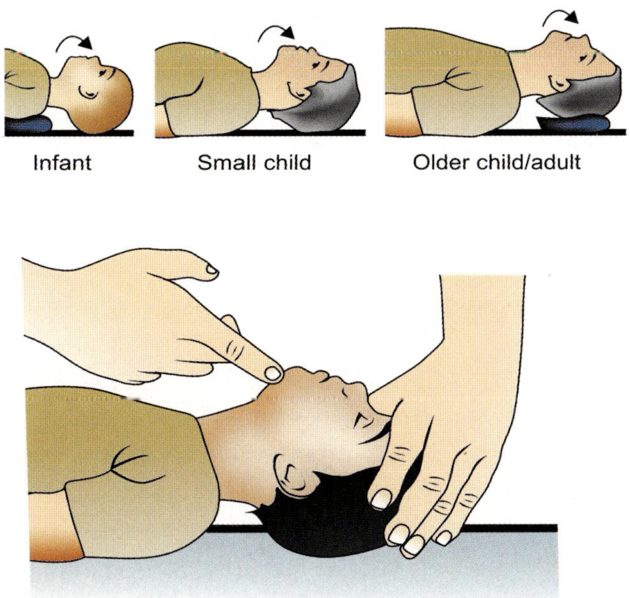

Fig. 5.6: Opening airway

Head tilt: place your hand on victim's forehead and gently tilt his head back.

Chin lift: lift the chin with your finger tips under the point of child's chin.

For mouth-to-mouth ventilation, pinch the soft part of the nose with index finger and thumb of the hand holding the victim's forehead. Allow mouth to open, but maintain chin lift. Take a breath and place your lips around the mouth with a good seal. Blow steadily into the mouth over one second watching for chest rise. Maintain head tilt and chin lift, take your mouth away and watch for chest to fall as air comes out. Repeat this sequence once more.

Infant

Neutral position of head and chin lift opens the airway. Take a breath and place your lips covering the mouth and nose of the infant with a good seal (mouth-to-mouth and nose technique). In older infants, attempt to seal only nose or mouth (keeping the other closed to prevent air escape), i.e. mouth-to-mouth or mouth to nose technique.

Each breath should be effective, i.e. chest rises and takes about one second. If the chest does not rise, reposition the head, try a better seal and attempt again for effective rescue breathing. Avoid excess ventilation.

Gastric inflation interferes with effective ventilation and causes regurgitation. Steps to minimize gastric inflation:

a. Avoid excess peak inspiration pressure by delivering only enough tidal volume for visible chest rise over approximately one second
b. Cricoid pressure (only in unresponsive victim and if additional HCP available), excess pressure may impede ventilation or speed or ease of intubation.
c. Passing a nasogastric/orogastric tube to relieve gastric inflation, especially if oxygenation and ventilation are compromised. Pass it after intubation as it interferes with gastroesophageal sphincter function and keep it open during ventilation.

Oxygen: Use 100% oxygen during resuscitation. Once ROSC is achieved FiO_2 should be titrated to minimum to achieve transcutaneous or arterial O_2 saturation of at least 94% to limit the risk of hyperoxemia while ensuring adequate oxygen delivery. (Oxygen saturation of 100% may correspond to a PaO_2 of 80-500 mm Hg, whereas SaO_2 of 94% ensures a PaO_2 of around 80 mm Hg). Whenever possible, oxygen should be humidified to prevent mucosal drying and thickening of pulmonary secretions. A simple oxygen mask can provide O_2 concentration of 30 to 50% in spontaneously breathing patient. A tight fitting nonrebreathing mask with oxygen inflow of 15 liters/ min maintains inflation of reservoir bag and a higher concentration of oxygen. Infant and pediatric size nasal cannulae provide oxygen concentration depending on child's size, respiration rate and respiratory effort.

BREATHING ADJUNCTS

- Barrier devices have not reduced the low risk of transmission of infection, and some may increase resistance to airflow.
- Bag and mask ventilation (BMV) is an essential CPR skill for a HCP, which requires training and periodic re-training for selecting the appropriate mask size, opening the airway, providing a tight seal between mask and face, delivering effective ventilation and assessing effectiveness of that ventilation (i.e. chest rise). Because of its complex steps, BMV is recommended only during 2 person CPR and even lone HCP should use mouth to barrier device technique instead of BMV. The self inflating bag should be at least 450–500 ml for infants and young children; an adult self-inflating bag (1000 ml) is used in older children, for effective ventilation.

- A self inflating bag delivers only room air (i.e. 21% oxygen) and when attached to O_2 inflow of 10 L/min, delivers O_2 in air up to 30-80% (also affected by tidal volume and peak inspiratory flow rate). To deliver a high O_2 concentration (60-95%), an O_2 reservoir bag should be attached with O_2 flow of 10-15 L/min (pediatric bag) and a flow of at least 15 L/min into an adult bag.
- Excessive ventilation by HCP is possible and particularly with advanced airway in place. It is harmful because it:
  - Increases intrathoracic pressure and impedes venous return, thereby decreases cardiac output which leads to cerebral and coronary hypoperfusion.
  - Causes air trapping and barotrauma in small air way obstruction, increases risk of regurgitation and aspiration.
- Use only the force and tidal volume necessary for slow visible chest rise over approximately one second. If the chest does not rise, re-do each step and then re-attempt ventilation.
- Two person BMV (one opens the airway with both hands and maintains the seal and the other compresses the ventilation bag) may be more effective than a single person technique in case of difficulty in creating a tight seal or when higher inspiration pressure is required as in case of significant airway obstruction or poor lung compliance.

DEFIBRILLATION

It is the definitive treatment for life-threatening cardiac arrhythmias such as VF and pulseless VT. Defibrillation consists of delivering a therapeutic dose of electrical energy to the affected heart which depolarizes a critical mass of heart muscle, terminates the arrhythmia and allows normal sinus rhythm to be re-established by the natural pacemaker, the SA node.

Non-shockable rhythms such as asystole and PEA (bradycardia with a wide QRS without palpable pulse) are most common in asphyxial arrest but VF is more likely in older children with sudden witnessed arrest. Thus in a witnessed sudden arrest AED should be used as soon as available whereas in an unwitnessed arrest 5 cycles or 2 minutes of CPR should be performed before using AED.

Defibrillators for resuscitation are either manual or automated (AED) with monophasic or biphasic waveforms **(Figs 5.7A and B)**. Many AEDs have specificity to recognize pediatric shockable rhythm (VF/pulseless VT) and to attenuate the delivered energy to 50-75 J for infants and children <25 kg or <8 yr of age. For infants, a manual defibrillator is preferred when a shockable rhythm is diagnosed by HCP. If neither defibrillator or AED is available, an unmodified adult AED may be used in infants with minimal myocardial damage and good neurological outcomes.

Infant paddles may slide over or are located under the adult paddles. Self-adhesive pads (hands-free) are also equally effective as paddles. Use the largest paddles or self-adhering electrodes possible on child's chest with a gap of 3 cm between them.

- Adult size for children >10 kg
- Infant size for infants <10 kg.

Electrode gel should be the interface between electrode and chest wall. Do not use saline-soaked pads, ultrasound gel, bare paddles or alcohol pads. The sternum electrode is placed over right side of upper chest to the right of the sternum and the apex electrode is over left lower ribs to the left of the nipple so that the heart is in between them. Connect the cables to the pads and AED.

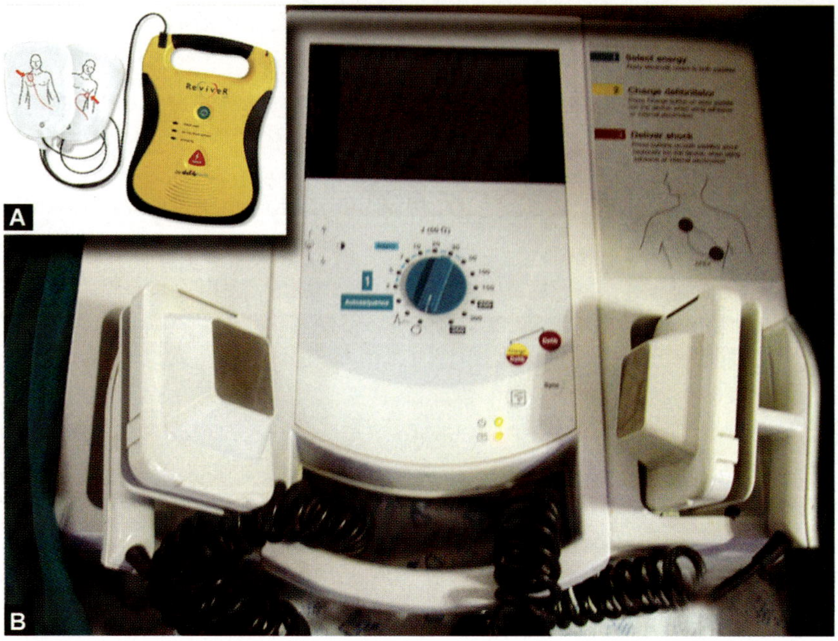

Figs 5.7A and B: (A) Automated external defibrillator; (B) Manual defibrillator

Energy dose: Biphasic shocks are as effective as monophasic shocks, but less harmful. Initial dose is 2 J/kg and subsequent dose should be at least 4 J/kg or higher (not to exceed 10 J/kg or adult maximum dose, whichever is lower), regardless of the type of defibrillator.

INTEGRATION OF DEFIBRILLATION SEQUENCE WITH RESUSCITATION SEQUENCE

1. Provide CPR until the defibrillator is available, defibrillation is more likely to be successful after a period of effective chest compression.
2. Chest compression is interrupted for rhythm check (by HCP from ECG or AED prompts).
3. Resume compression after a rhythm check while the defibrillator is charging.
4. End CPR cycle with compression for shock delivery and minimize time interval between compression and shock delivery and resumption of chest compression after shock delivery.
5. If first shock (2 J/kg) is ineffective, resumption of CPR for 2 minutes is of greater value than another immediate shock. CPR provides coronary perfusion, increasing the likelihood of successful defibrillation with a subsequent shock (4 J/kg or higher).
6. If rhythm becomes unshockable, continue with asystole or PEA algorithm.
7. If second shock is ineffective, continue with CPR for 2 minutes with epinephrine dose and shock subsequently. If still unsuccessful, while continuing CPR, give amiodarone or lidocaine if amiodarone is not available.
8. If defibrillation successfully restores a perfusing rhythm with palpable pulse, continue with post resuscitation care.
9. If defibrillation is successful, but subsequently VF recurs, resume CPR and give another bolus of amiodarone before attempting defibrillation with the previously successful shock dose.
10. Search for and treat reversible causes.

BLS Sequence for Lay Rescuer

AHA–BLS guidelines delineate a series of skills traditionally described as a sequence of distinct steps which are meant for true for a lone rescuer, but should be performed simultaneously in case more than one rescuer is present.

a. *Safety of the rescuer and victim:* First and foremost, the safety of the rescuer and victim should be ensured. The victim should be moved only if the area is not safe. CPR carries a theoretical risk of transmitting infectious disease, though the risk to the rescuer is very low.
b. *Assess the need for CPR:* A lay rescuer should assume that cardiac arrest is present if the victim is unresponsive and not breathing or only gasping.
   - *Check for response:* Gently tap the victim and call the child's name (if you know it). Ask loudly – "Are you alright?" If the child responds by moving, moaning or answering, quickly check for any injury that needs medical assistance. In case of a lone rescuer and victim is breathing, leave the child to phone the ERS, but return quickly and reassess his condition frequently. Children with respiratory distress may assume a position that maintains airway patency with optimal ventilation. Allow such children to remain in that comfortable position. If the child is unresponsive, shout for help.
   - *Check for breathing:* In case of regular breathing and no evidence of trauma, turn the child onto his side in recovery position for a patent airway and decreased aspiration risk. He does not need CPR.

   If unresponsive and gasping or not breathing regularly, begin CPR. The gasps or infrequent, irregular breaths should be treated as a situation of apnea.
c. Start high-quality chest compressions
d. Open airway and give ventilations

   Compression to ventilation ratio is 30:2.
   - The lone rescuer should give five cycles of 30:2 compressions and ventilation in 2 minutes before leaving to activate the ERS and obtain an AED if one is available nearby.
   - In case of two rescuers, one should start CPR immediately while the other activates ERS and obtains AED if available.
   - Attach ECG monitors or AED pads as soon as available.

BLS Sequence for Health Care Provider (HCP)

Since HCPs are less likely to be lone rescuers, individual steps are often performed simultaneously (less significant which is performed first). It is reasonable to tailor the sequence of rescue actions to the most likely causes of arrest **(Fig. 5.8)**.

Pulse check: If the victim is unresponsive and gasping or not breathing, attempt to feel for a pulse within 10 seconds (brachial pulse in infant, carotid or femoral pulse in a child).

a. If not sure of a pulse within 10 sec, begin chest compression.
b. If palpable pulse $\geq$ 60 per minute but inadequate breathing, give rescue breaths at the rate of 12-20 breaths per minute (1 breath every 3-5 sec) until spontaneous breathing resumes. Reassess pulse every 2 minutes, but do not spend more than 10 sec on it.
c. If palpable pulse < 60 per minute with signs of poor perfusion (i.e. pallor, mottling, cyanosis) despite support of oxygenation and ventilation, begin chest compression because cardiac output in children largely depends on heart rate. Profound bradycardia with poor

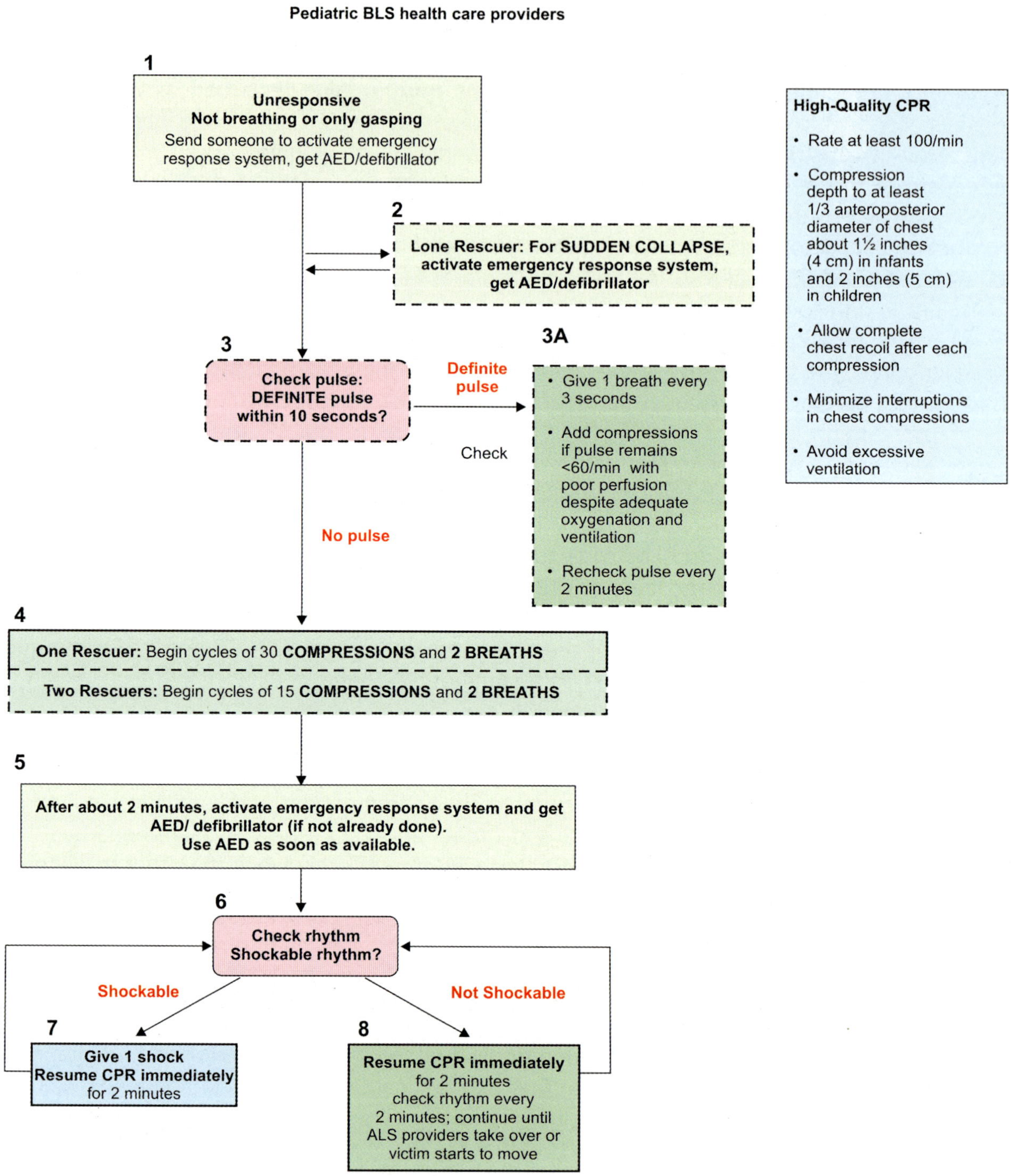

Note: The boxes bordered with dashed lines are performed by health care providers and not by lay resuers

Fig. 5.8: Pediatric BLS algorithm. (Reproduced with permission from Pediatrics. American Academy of Pediatrics. 2010;126:e1349)

perfusion precedes imminent cardiac arrest and CPR prior to full cardiac arrest leads to the best survival (64%) to discharge.

CHEST COMPRESSION

The only difference from sequence for lay rescuers is that the technique for infants is 2-thumb-encircling hands technique when more than one rescuer is present.

VENTILATION

Lone rescuer—compression:ventilation = 30:2
Two rescuers—compression:ventilation = 15:2

In case of suspected spinal injury, use jaw thrust without head-tilt to open the airway. Since a patent airway and adequate ventilation is important in pediatric CPR, use a head tilt – chin lift maneuver if the jaw thrust does not open the airway. If an advanced airway is in place, the compressing rescuer delivers continuously without pause for ventilation. The ventilation rescuer delivers 8-10 breaths per minute (breath every 6-8 sec) without interrupting chest compression.

Pediatric Advanced Life Support (PALS)

PALS usually takes place as a rapid organized response in an advanced health care environment by multiple responders in the form of simultaneous coordinated steps. While one rescuer performs chest compressions, another performs ventilation and other rescuer should obtain a monitor/defibrillator, establish vascular access and calculate and prepare the anticipated medication **(Fig. 5.9)**.

Common reasons for not performing high quality CPR:

- Rescuer inattention to details
- Rescuer fatigue
- Long or frequent interruptions to secure airway, check cardiac rhythm and transfer the patient.

In the ICU, the waveform of an indwelling arterial catheter helps to evaluate hand position and chest compression depth. A minor adjustment of hand position or depth of compression can significantly improve the amplitude of arterial waveform reflecting better chest compression induced stroke volume. The arterial waveform also identifies ROSC. Monitoring exhaled CO_2, ideally by capnography confirms correct ETT position and also gives an indication of ROSC (abrupt and sustained rise in $EtCO_2$). If the $EtCO_2$ is consistently < 10-15 mm Hg, focus on improving the chest compression quality and avoid excessive ventilation. $EtCO_2$ must be interpreted with caution for 1-2 minutes after intravenous bolus of epinephrine or any vasoconstrictive medications because these medications may transiently decrease the pulmonary blood flow and exhaled CO_2 below the limits of detection. Severe airway obstruction (e.g. status asthmaticus) and pulmonary edema may impair CO_2 elimination below the limit of detection. A large glottic air leak also may reduce exhaled tidal volume through ETT and dilute CO_2 concentration. Echocardiography may be considered to identify patients with potentially treatable causes of arrest, particularly pericardial tamponade and inadequate ventricular filling. Minimize interruptions in CPR while performing echocardiography.

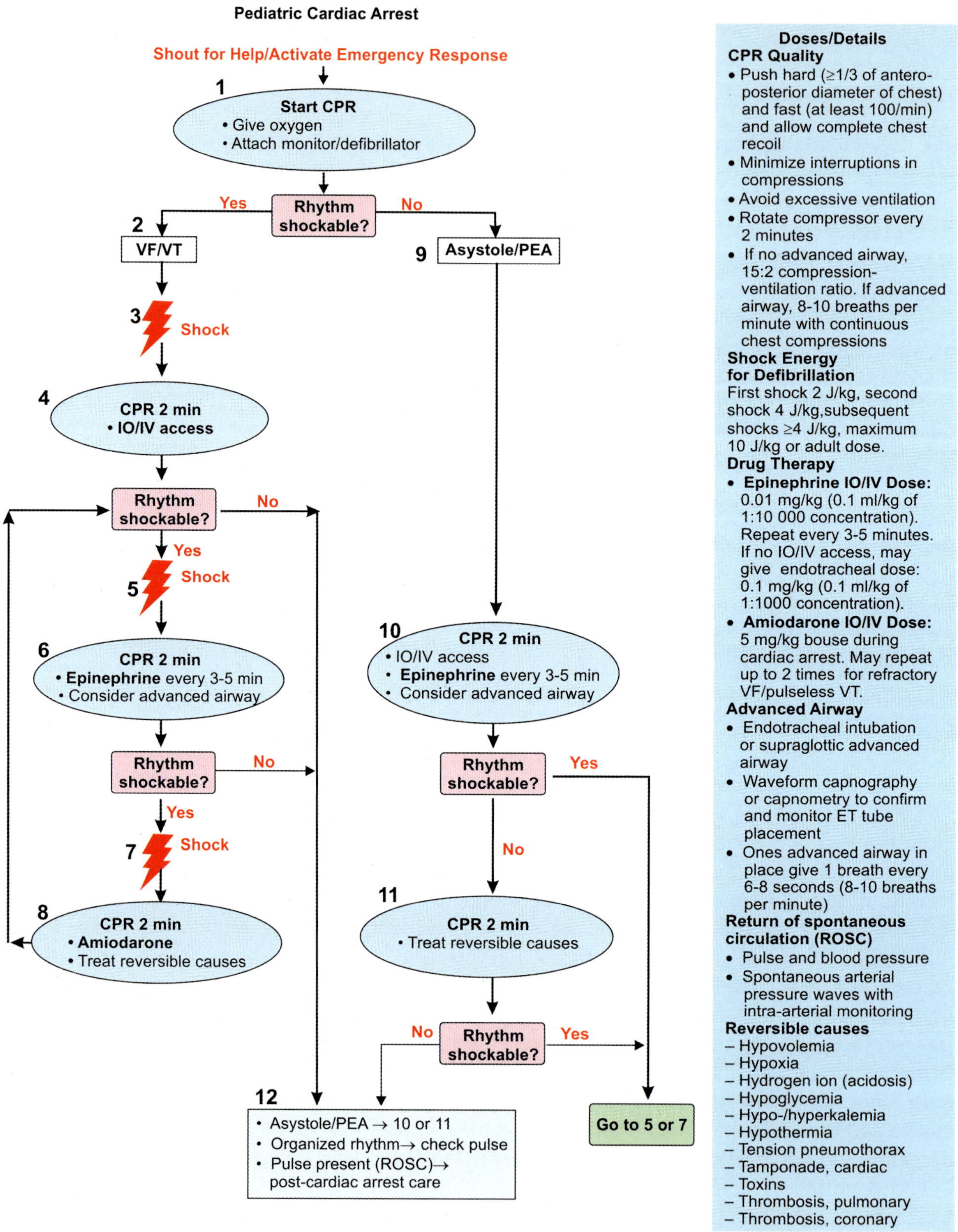

Fig. 5.9: Pediatric cardiac arrest. (Reproduced with permission from Pediatrics. American Academy of Pediatrics. 2010;126:e1371)

Emergency Fluids and Medications

The child's actual body weight is used for calculating the initial resuscitation drug doses. However, in out-of- hospital setting and obese children, body length tape with pre-calculated doses is clinically validated and has been proved to be more accurate than age-based or observer's estimate based methods in prediction of body weight.

For subsequent doses of resuscitation drugs in both obese and nonobese patients, the PALS providers may consider adjusting doses to achieve the desired therapeutic level. However, it should never exceed the standard dose for adults.

VASCULAR ACCESS

Vascular access is essential during resuscitation for administration of medications and drawing blood samples. Peripheral venous access in children can be challenging during an emergency. Central venous line provides more secure long-term venous access but its placement is time consuming. Central drug administration does not achieve higher drug levels or a more rapid response than peripheral administration. Limit the time spent in attempting venous access in a critically ill child. Intraosseous (IO) access is a rapid, safe and effective route for administration of fluids, drugs and to obtain an initial blood sample during resuscitation. Onset of action and drug levels following IO infusion during CPR are comparable to those achieved following vascular administration. Use manual pressure or infusion pump to inject viscous drugs or rapid fluid boluses. Follow each bolus injection with a saline flush to promote entry into central circulation.

ENDOTRACHEAL ROUTE

If IV or IO route is not possible, lipid soluble drugs such as lignocaine, epinephrine, atropine and naloxone (LEAN) can be given via ETT. Optimum dose by this route is not known but lower blood concentrations are achieved than the same dose given intravenously. Drugs should be flushed by 5 ml of normal saline followed by 5 assisted breaths. Nonlipid-soluble drugs like sodium bicarbonate and calcium may injure the airway and should not be given by this route.

FLUIDS

Lactated ringer's solution or normal saline are the fluids of choice for initial resuscitation. Bolus of glucose containing fluids should only be given in documented hypoglycemia. There is no benefit in using colloid as initial fluid.

MEDICATIONS (TABLE 5.1)

Adenosine

It causes a temporary atrioventricular nodal conduction block and interrupts reentry circuits that involve AV node. Its short half-life provides a wide margin of safety. It should always be administered as close to the heart as possible followed by a rapid saline flush to promote drug delivery.

Amiodarone

It slows AV conduction, prolongs AV refractory period and QT interval and slows ventricular conduction (widens QRS). Expert consultation is strongly recommended prior to its use in a pediatric patient with a perfusing rhythm. The severity of hypotension due to its vasodilator

Table 5.1: Medications for pediatric resuscitation and arrhythmia

Drug	*Dose (IV/IO)*	*Maximum dose*	*Considerations*
Adenosine	0.1 mg kg^{-1} 0.2 mg kg^{-1} (Second dose)	6 mg 12 mg	Rapid bolus with flush Monitor ECG
Amiodarone	5 mg kg^{-1} over 30 min	300 mg	Repeat upto maximum total dose of 15 mg kg^{-1} Monitor ECG, blood pressure Bolus dose only during arrest
Atropine	0.02 mg kg^{-1}	0.5 mg	Repeat once if needed Minimum IV dose: 0.1 mg Endotracheal dose 2-3 times higher
Calcium chloride	20 mg kg^{-1}	2 gm	Slow administration
Epinephrine	0.01 mg kg^{-1} (1:10,000) Endotracheal route: 0.1 mg kg^{-1} (1:1000)	1 mg 2.5 mg	Repeated every 3-5 minutes Low dose harmful because of β-vasodilatation High dose harmful too except in β-blocker overdosage
Glucose	0.5-1 gm kg^{-1}		10% Dextrose: 5-10 ml kg^{-1} (newborn) 25% Dextrose: 2-5 ml kg^{-1} (infant, children) 50% Dextrose: 1-2 ml kg^{-1} (adolescent)
Lidocaine	1 mg kg^{-1} followed by 20-50 mg kg^{-1} min^{-1}		
Magnesium sulfate	25-50 mg kg^{-1}	2 gm	Slowly inject over 10-20 min Inject faster in torsades de pointes
Naloxone	0.1 mg kg^{-1} < 5 yrs/20 kg 2 mg $\geq$ 5 yrs/20 kg		Lower doses (1-5 μg kg^{-1}) to reverse respiratory depression related to therapeutic opioid use
Procainamide	15 mg kg^{-1} over 30-60 min		Monitor ECG and blood pressure
Sodium bicarbonate	1 mEq kg^{-1}		Used after establishing adequate ventilation
Verapamil	0.1-0.3 mg kg^{-1}		Only for SVT in older children Restricted use in infants Potential myocardial depression, hypotension and cardiac arrest

property is related to the infusion rate. The infusion is slowed if there is prolongation of QT interval of heart block and stopped if QRS widens to > 50% of base line or hypotension occurs. Other potential complications are bradycardia and torsades de pointes VT. Its adverse effects are long lasting as amiodarone's half life is upto 40 days.

Atropine

It is a parasympatholytic drug that accelerates sinus or atrial pacemaker and increases AV conduction. Small doses (<0.1 mg) may produce paradoxical bradycardia because of its central effect. It is indicated in the treatment of asystole, bradycardia with hypotension, second and third degree heart block.

Calcium

Routine calcium administration is not recommended as it has no benefit and may be harmful. It is only indicated in case of documented hypocalcemia, hyperkalemia, hypermagnesemia and calcium channel blocker overdose. In case of peripheral venous access and nonarrest setting, calcium gluconate is recommended because of its lower osmolality than calcium chloride.

In critically ill children, calcium chloride may be preferred because of the greater availability of ionized calcium.

Epinephrine

It has both potent α- and β- adrenergic effects. At low doses, the β-adrenergic effects may predominate, leading to decreased SVR, but the α adrenergic mediated vasconstriction predominates in the dose used during cardiac arrest, thus increasing aortic diastolic pressure and coronary perfusion, a critical determinant of successful resuscitation from cardiac arrest. It should not be administered simultaneously in the same tubing with sodium bicarbonate as the alkaline solution inactivates epinephrine. In children with perfusing rhythm, epinephrine can cause tachyarrhythmias, ventricular ectopy and hypertension.

Glucose

Infants have a relatively high glucose requirement and low glycogen store. Therefore, they are likely to develop hypoglycemia. Check blood glucose level during resuscitation and treat hypoglycemia.

Lidocaine

It decreases automaticity and suppresses ventricular arrhythmia, but less effective than amiodarone for improving ROSC in VF refractory to shocks and epinephrine. Its toxicity includes myocardial and circulatory depression, drowsiness, disorientation, muscle twitching and seizures, especially in states of poor cardiac output and hepatic or renal failure.

Magnesium

It is indicated for the treatment of documented hypomagnesemia or for torsades de pointes (polymorphic VT with long QT interval). Rapid administration causes vasodilation and hypotension.

Procainamide

It prolongs the refractory period of the atria and ventricles and depresses conduction velocity. The precautions during administration are the same as that for amiodarone.

Sodium Bicarbonate

Routine administration during cardiac arrest is not recommended. It may be indicated in some toxidromes (i.e. tricyclic antidepressant overdose) or special resuscitation situations such as hyperkalemic cardiac arrest . During severe shock or cardiac arrest, ABG analysis may not accurately reflect tissue and venous acidosis. Excess sodium bicarbonate may impair tissue oxygen delivery, cause hypokalemia, hypocalcemia, hypernatremia and hyperosmolality, decreases the VF threshold and impair cardiac function.

Post-resuscitation Stabilization

OBJECTIVES

- To preserve neurologic function
- To limit secondary organ injury
- To diagnose and treat the cause of illness
- To reach a pediatric tertiary care center in an optimal physiological state.

APPROACH

Frequent reassessment is necessary because cardiorespiratory status may deteriorate at any time:

1. Hyperventilation should be avoided as it may impair neurological outcome by adversely affecting cardiac output and thereby cerebral perfusion. However, brief periods of hyperventilation may be advised as temporary rescue therapy in the scenario of impending cerebral herniation (e.g. sudden rise in intracranial pressure, non-reactive dilated pupils, bradycardia, hypertension).
2. Use the lowest inspired oxygen concentration that will maintain the arterial oxyhemoglobin saturation $\geq$94% and avoid hyperoxemia which causes oxidative injury following ischemia reperfusion.
3. Induced therapeutic hypothermia (32°C-34°C) may be beneficial for infants and children who remain comatose after resuscitation; and adolescents who remain comatose after resuscitation from sudden, witnessed, out-of-hospital VF cardiac arrest. Prevent shivering by sedation and/or neuromuscular blockade (it may mask seizure activity). Potential complications of hypothermia include infection, arrhythmia, diminished cardiac output, thrombocytopenia, coagulopathy, hypovolemia, hypokalemia, hypomagnesemia. Avoid rewarming faster than 0.5°C per 2 hours unless clinically indicated.
4. Fever >38°C should be treated aggressively with antipyretics and cooling devices along with temperature monitoring, because fever adversely influences recovery from ischemic brain injury.
5. Post-ischemic seizures should be aggressively treated and if possible, the correctable metabolic causes such as hypoglycemia or dyselectrolytemia should be rectified.
6. In case of significant respiratory compromise (i.e. tachypnea, respiratory distress, agitation, cyanosis, hypoxemia), ventilation should be assisted. If already intubated, the position and patency of ETT should be verified. ABG should be evaluated after 10-15 mins of mechanical ventilation and appropriate adjustments in ventilator settings should be done.
7. Resolution of metabolic acidosis, reduction in lactate level and normalization of venous oxygen saturation indicate adequate tissue perfusion and oxygenation.
8. Analgesics, sedatives and neuromuscular blockers play an important role in improving oxygenation and ventilation in case of painful conditions or patient-ventilator dysynchrony or severely compromised pulmonary function.
9. Monitor heart-rate, blood pressure, exhaled CO_2, urine output and venous or arterial blood gas analysis and serum electrolytes, glucose and calcium. Clinical evaluation should be repeated at frequent intervals until the patient is stable. Decreased urine output (< 1 ml/kg/hr in infants and children or <30 ml/hr in adolescents) may be caused by pre-renal (dehydration, hypotension) or renal ischemic damage or both. Avoid nephrotoxic medications and adjust the dose of medications excreted by the kidneys until renal function is estimated.
10. Myocardial dysfunction with vascular instability is common following resuscitation from cardiac arrest. There is an initial hyperdynamic state replaced by worsening cardiac function over time. Systemic and pulmonary vascular resistances are often increased initially except in some cases of septic shock. Therefore, it is recommended to start vasoactive drugs in a titrated dose to improve myocardial function and organ perfusion in infants and children with documented or suspected cardiovascular dysfunction after cardiac arrest **(Table 5.2)**. There is great interpatient variability in response, therefore, each drug and dose should be tailored to the desired effect. The vasoactive drugs should always be administered into a

Table 5.2: Vasoactive drugs used in post-resuscitation phase

Epinephrine	0.1-1 μg kg^{-1} min^{-1} IV/IO	< 0.3 μg kg^{-1} min^{-1} → β adrenergic actions (tachycardia, inotropy, ↓ SVR) > 0.3 μg kg^{-1} min^{-1} → α-adrenergic vasoconstriction
Norepinephrine	0.1-2 μg kg^{-1} min^{-1}	Potent vasopressor Used in shock unresponsive to fluid and low SVR (i.e. septic, anaphylactic, spinal, vasodilatory shock)
Dopamine	2-20 μg kg^{-1} min^{-1} IV/IO	< 5 mcg kg^{-1} min^{-1} → Low dose – direct dopaminergic effect > 5 mcg kg^{-1} min^{-1} → High dose – cardiac β-stimulation (less effect in infant or chronic CCF) > 20 mcg kg^{-1} min^{-1} → α-adrenergic effect – excess vasoconstriction
Dobutamine	2-20 μg kg^{-1} min^{-1} IV/IO	Selective β_1 and β_2 action – Inotrope, vasodilator Use in low CO states due to myocardial dysfunction
Sodium nitroprusside	0.5-8 μg kg^{-1} min^{-1}	Reduces afterload, ↑ CO in case of poor myocardial function Needs to be used with an inotrope Fluid is required secondary to vasodilatory effect.
Milrinone	50 μg kg^{-1} IV/IO over 10-60 min then 0.25-0.75 μg kg^{-1} min^{-1}	Inodilator action with little effect on myocardial oxygen demand Effective in increased systemic and pulmonary vascular resistance

secure IV line. Epinephrine or norepinephrine may be preferable to dopamine especially in infants with marked circulatory instability and decompensated shock.

There is increasing evidence that some cases of sudden, unexplained deaths in infants and children may be associated with genetic mutations that cause cardiac ion transport defects (i.e. channelopathies). They can cause fatal arrhythmia and their correct diagnosis may be critically important for living relatives. So a complete past medical and family history, review of previous ECGs and genetic analysis of tissues should be evaluated for aid in diagnosis.

Major Changes Introduced in 2010 CPR Guidelines

1. Whenever possible, the family members should have the option of being present during resuscitation as it helps them to deal with the inevitable trauma and grief following the death of a child.
2. Integrated post-cardiac arrest care has been added as the fifth link to the AHA pediatric chain of survival.
3. Early recognition of cardiac arrest is essential as CPR is the only treatment for sudden cardiac arrest. Action is emphasized instead of assessment, i.e. "look-listen-feel for breathing" sequence is removed from algorithm. Start CPR and call ERS the moment you realize that the victim is unresponsive and not breathing.
4. De-emphasis of pulse check for HCP: if a pulse can not be detected within 10 seconds, HCP should begin CPR.
   Reason: There is evidence that HCP can not reliably and rapidly detect either presence or absence of a pulse. Given the risk of not providing chest compressions for a cardiac arrest victim and relatively minimal risk of providing chest compressions when a pulse is present, it is recommended to start CPR if HCP is unsure about the pulse.
5. Three steps of CPR have been rearranged as C-A-B instead of A-B-C, the only exception being neonatal CPR, because chest compression is a priority before worrying about airway.

6. High quality chest compression is emphasized.
   The absolute depth of compression is deeper than in previous guidelines. CV ratio of 30:2 yields more chest compression than a 15:2 ratio with minimal or no increase in rescuer fatigue and less "no-flow" time. This universal CV ratio enables anyone trained in adult BLS to resuscitate children with minimal additional information. As ventilation remains a very important component of CPR in asphyxial arrest, CV ratio of 15:2 is preferable when more than one rescuer is available in case of HCP.
7. Hands-only CPR or Compression-only CPR should be continued till help arrives if the rescuer is unable or unwilling to give rescue breathing.
   Reason: Resuscitation outcomes in infants and children are best if chest compression is combined with ventilation, but compression alone is preferable to no CPR
8. Defibrillation may be used in infants
9. Monitoring exhaled CO_2 detection (capnography or colorimetry) is recommended whenever ETT is placed with a perfusing cardiac rhythm as well as during CPR to assess and optimize quality of chest compressions.
10. Once ROSC is achieved, adjust FiO_2 to reduce PaO_2 to normal levels to reduce the risk of oxidative injury by hyperoxia.
11. QRS width > 0.09 seconds (instead of > 0.08 seconds in 2005 guidelines) is considered as wide complex tachycardia.
12. Recommendations for specific resuscitation guidance have been added to the management of cardiac arrest in infants and children with single-ventricle anatomy, Fontan or hemi-Fontan bidirectional Glenn physiology and pulmonary hypertension. Early use of extracorporeal membrane oxygenation as rescue therapy in centers with this advanced facility is common in all these scenarios.

Foreign Body Airway Obstruction (FBAO)

More than 90% of childhood deaths from foreign body aspiration occur in children less than 5 years of age; 65% of the victims are infants. The most common cause of choking is liquid in infants and small objects or food items like candies, nuts, grapes, etc. in children.

DIAGNOSIS

Signs of FBAO include a sudden onset of respiratory distress with coughing, gagging, stridor or wheezing, cyanosis and unconsciousness (if airway obstruction not relieved immediately). Absence of fever and congestion differentiates it from infectious cause such as croup. Older children may exhibit universal choking sign of clutching his neck with thumb and index finger.

MANAGEMENT (FIG. 5.10)

a. *Mild obstruction:* The child is conscious, can cough and make some sounds. Do not interfere, allow the victim to clear the airway by coughing forcefully while you observe for signs of severe FBAO (i.e. poor ineffective cough, stridor, cyanosis and loss of consciousness).
b. *Severe obstruction:* The victim can not cough or make any sound.

In case of a child who is conscious and standing, perform subdiaphragmatic abdominal thrusts (Heimlich maneuver) until object is expelled or victim becomes unresponsive. Steps of Heimlich maneuver which forces air from victim's lungs and expel the foreign body are as follows **(Fig. 5.11):**

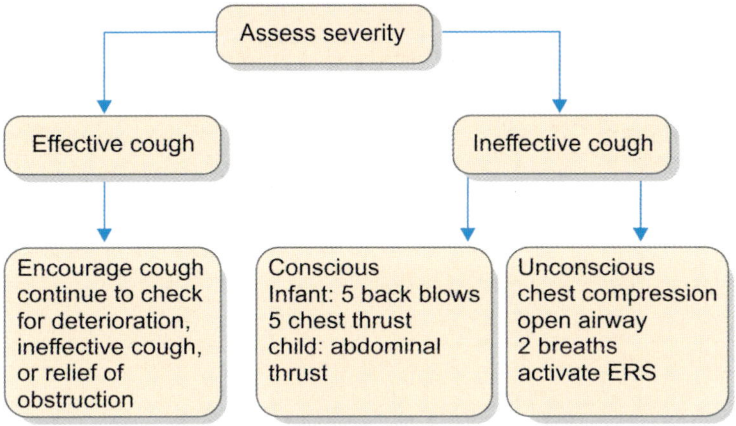

Fig. 5.10: Pediatric FBAO treatment

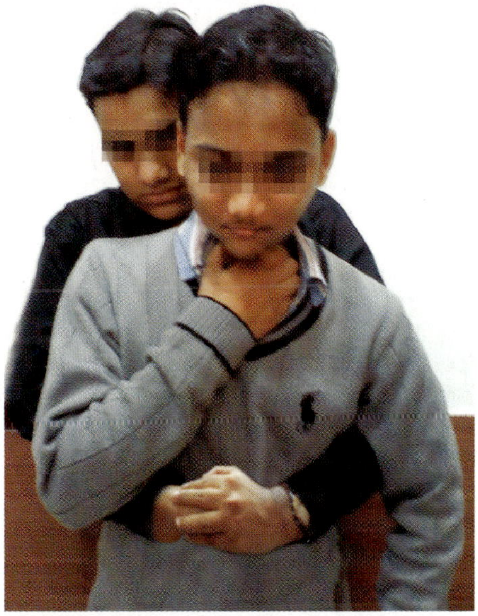

Fig. 5.11: Heimlich maneuver

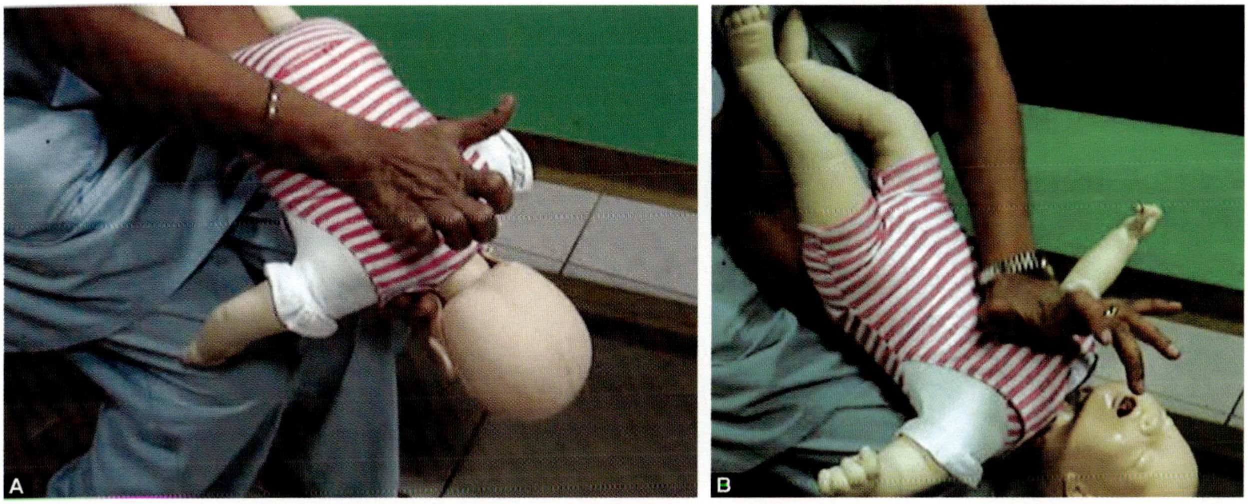

Figs 5.12A and B: (A) Back slap (infant); (B) Chest compression (infant)

- Make a fist with one hand.
- Place the thumb side of the fist on the victim's abdomen just above the umbilicus and well below the xiphisternum.
- Grasp the fist with the other hand and provide quick upward thrusts into the victim's abdomen.

For an infant, straddle the infant prone on your arm and deliver repeated cycles of 5 back blows (slaps) followed by 5 chest compressions in supine position until the object is expelled or victim becomes unresponsive **(Figs 5.12A and B)**. Abdominal thrusts are not recommended because of possible damage to relatively large and unprotected liver (due to horizontal ribs). If the infant becomes unresponsive, place him flat on the back, start CPR with chest compressions (no pulse check is required). After 30 chest compressions, open the airway. If you see a FB, remove it but a blind finger sweep is not advisable because it may push obstructing objects farther into the pharynx and may damage the oropharynx. Attempt to give 2 breaths and continue with cycles of chest compressions and ventilations until the object is expelled. After 2 minutes of CPR, activate ERS.

6 Neonatal Resuscitation

Successful neonatal resuscitation requires:

- Understanding of fetal-neonatal physiology and its adaptation to extrauterine life
- Acquisition and maintenance of proper resuscitative equipment and medication
- Anticipating the need for resuscitation, accurate evaluation and prompt initiation of support.

The goal of guidelines for neonatal resuscitation issued by the American Heart Association (AHA) and American Academy of Pediatrics (AAP) is to prevent the morbidity and mortality associated with hypoxic-ischemic tissue (brain, heart, kidney) injury and to re-establish adequate spontaneous respiration and cardiac output **(Fig. 6.1)**.

Approximately 10% of newborns require some assistance to begin breathing at birth and less than 1% require extensive resuscitation measures. The following resuscitative measures apply primarily to the newly born undergoing transition from intrauterine to extrauterine life, but are also applicable to neonates who have completed perinatal transition and require resuscitation during the first few weeks to months following birth. (The term 'newly born' apply to an infant at time of birth and the terms "newborn" and "neonate" apply to any infant during initial hospitalization).

The newly born infants who do not require resuscitation are generally identified by a rapid assessment of following three features:

1. Term gestation
2. Crying or breathing
3. Good muscle tone.

If the answer is "yes" to all the above 3 points, the baby should be dried, placed skin-to-skin with the mother and covered with dry linen to maintain temperature. Observation of breathing, activity and color should always be an ongoing process. There is increasing evidence of the benefit of delaying cord clamping for at least 1 minute in term and preterm infants not requiring resuscitation. There is insufficient evidence to support or refute to delay of cord clamping in babies requiring resuscitation.

If the answer is "no" to any of the above-mentioned three assessment features, the newly born is definitely in need of resuscitation measures.

Steps of Resuscitation

A. Initial steps in stabilization
B. Ventilation
C. Chest compression
D. Administration of epinephrine and/or volume expansion.

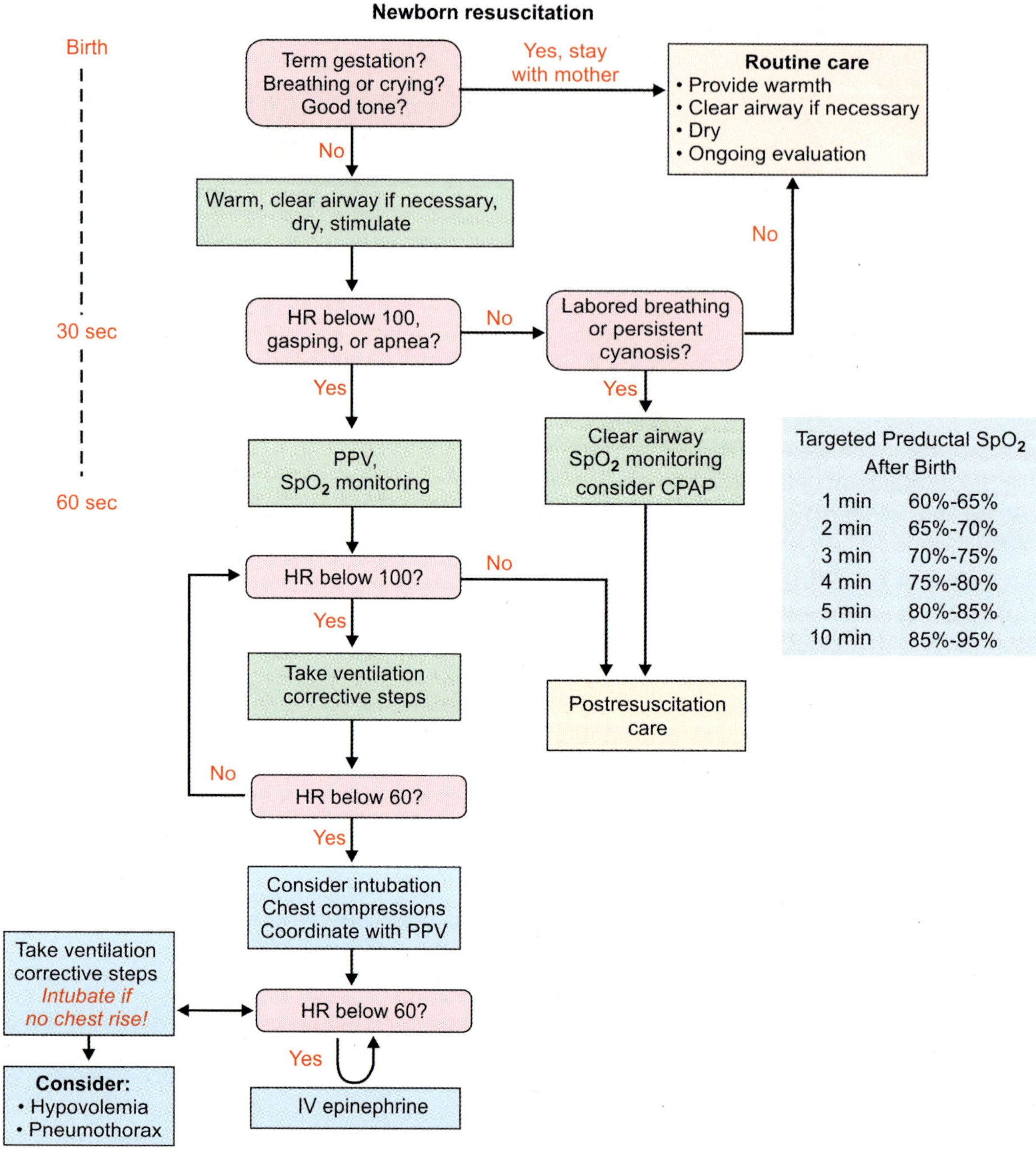

Fig. 6.1: Newborn resuscitation algorithm. (*Source:* John Kattwinkel, et al. Neonatal Resuscitation. Guidelines for Cardiopulmonary Resuscitation and Emergency Cardiovascular Care. 2010;122(18 suppl 3)

The decision to progress from one step to the next is determined by the simultaneous assessment of two vital signs, i.e. respiration and heart rate. At every delivery there should be at least one person available who is responsible only for the newly born and should be capable of initiating resuscitation, including administration of positive pressure ventilation (PPV) and chest compression. Either this person or someone else who is promptly available should have the skills of complete resuscitation including endotracheal intubation and administration of medications.

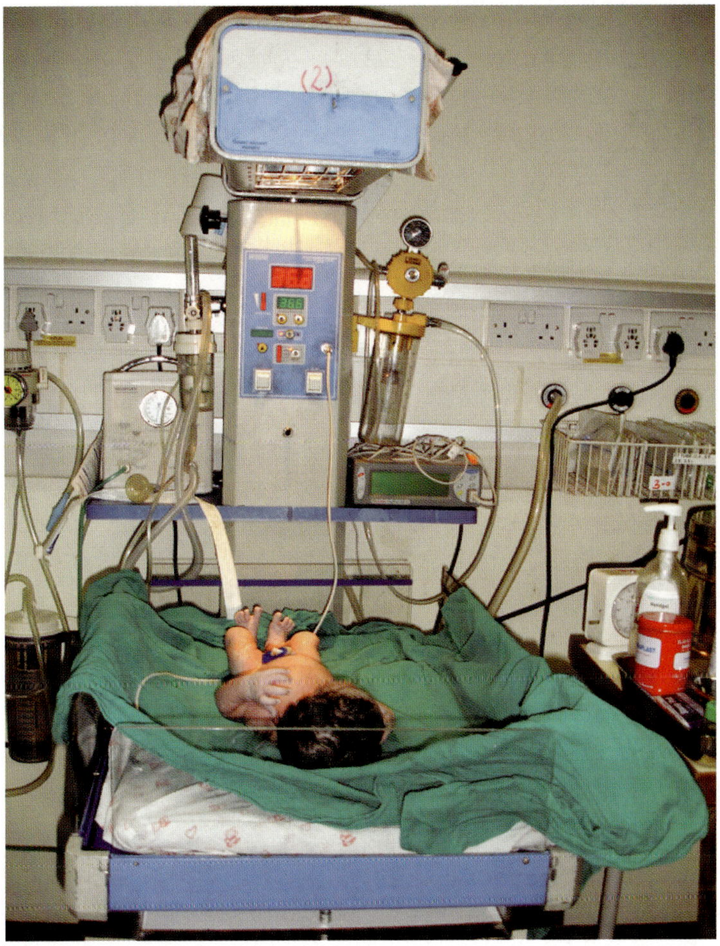

Fig. 6.2: Neonatal resuscitation trolley

High-risk births such as severe IUGR, preterm delivery, choanal atresia, pharyngeal airway malformations, laryngeal web, pneumothorax, pleural effusion and diaphragmatic hernia, etc. may require recruitment of additional skilled personnel for immediate interventions as required.

INITIAL STEPS IN STABILIZATION

Approximately 60 seconds ("the golden minute") is allotted for completing the initial steps, re-evaluating and beginning the next step (ventilation) if required **(Fig. 6.2)**.

- Provide warmth by placing the baby under a radiant heat source
- Position head in a "sniffing" position to open the airway
- Clear the airway if necessary with a bulb syringe or suction catheter
- Dry the baby and stimulate breathing.

Temperature Control

The goal is to achieve normothermia and avoid hypothermia or iatrogenic hyperthermia. Additional warming techniques are required to prevent hypothermia in extremely low birth weight (ELBW) babies (<1500 g) as their thin skin and large surface area contribute to rapid heat loss. The different warming techniques are:

- Increasing environmental temperature of delivery room to 26°C
- Food or medical grade, heat resistant plastic wrapping to cover the baby

- Placing the baby on warming mattress
- Prewarming the linen used to cover the baby
- Placing the baby skin-to-skin with mother and covering both with a blanket
- Placing the baby under radiant heat with servo-controlled temperature support.

All resuscitation procedures should be performed with these temperature controlling interventions in place. The infant's temperature must be closely monitored because hyperthermia remains a risk particularly when a combination of temperature control techniques is used. Avoiding hyperthermia is particularly important in infants who may have had a hypoxic-ischemic event.

Clearing the Airway

- Intrapartum suctioning (i.e. before delivery of shoulders) is not recommended
- In case of clear amniotic fluid, gentle suctioning of nasopharynx should be done after placing the baby under radiant warmer, only in babies who have obvious obstruction to spontaneous breathing or who require PPV
- In case of meconium-stained liquor, endotracheal intubation and suction of endotracheal tube while withdrawing it is recommended only if the baby is not active. However, in case of an unsuccessful or a prolonged attempt at intubation, bag and mask ventilation (BMV) should be considered, particularly if there is persistent bradycardia.

Rationale for Such Recommendations

a. Suctioning of nasopharynx can create bradycardia during resuscitation
b. Suctioning of the trachea in intubated babies receiving mechanical ventilation in neonatal intensive care unit (NICU) can be associated with a deterioration in pulmonary compliance and oxygenation and reduction in cerebral blood flow velocity when done routinely, even in the absence of obvious oral or nasal secretions.
c. Elective and routine endotracheal intubation and direct suctioning of the trachea have no added benefit in the case of meconium stained babies, who were vigorous at birth.

Oxygen Need and Administration

Assessment of oxygen need and administration of oxygen in neonatal resuscitation is particularly important because either insufficient or excessive oxygenation can be detrimental. Hypoxemia and ischemia cause injury to multiple organs whereas even brief exposure to excessive oxygen during and following resuscitation can trigger inflammatory responses and oxidative stress in newborn.

An uncompromised newly born will achieve and maintain pink mucous membrane without administration of supplementary oxygen, because the blood oxygen levels do not reach extrauterine values (>90%) until approximately 10 minutes following birth. Oxyhemoglobin saturation may normally remain in 70-80% range for several minutes following birth thus resulting in cyanosis during that period. Assessment of skin color or lack of cyanosis appears to be a very poor indicator of the state of oxyhemoglobin saturation or state of oxygenation of an uncompromised baby following birth.

The standard approach for resuscitation is to use air or blended oxygen to achieve SpO_2 in the target range **(Fig. 6.1)** guided by pulse oximetry. If there is severe bradycardia, i.e. heart rate less tha 60 beats per minute (bpm) after 90 seconds of resuscitation with lower concentration of oxygen, oxygen concentration should be increased to 100% until normal heart rate sets in.

In situations where supplemental oxygen is not readily available, PPV should be administered with room air.

Pulse oximetry should be used in anticipated resuscitation delivery of PPV for more than a few breaths, persistent cyanosis or when supplemental oxygen is administered. The oximeter probe should be attached to a pre-ductal location (i.e. right palm). Oximetry is reliable as long as there is sufficient cardiac output and skin blood flow.

POSITIVE PRESSURE VENTILATION

If the infant remains apneic or gasping or the heart rate remains <100 bpm after administering the initial steps, PPV is to be started.

- Assisted ventilation rates should be 40-60 breaths per minute
- An initial inflation pressure of 20 cm H_2O for 1 second may be effective, but 30-40 cm H_2O pressure may be required in some term babies without spontaneous respiration
- Preterm babies have immature lungs which are more difficult to ventilate and more prone to injury by large volume inflation during PPV. Thus the initial peak inflation pressure (PIP) should be individualized to achieve a prompt improvement in heart rate and to maintain it at > 100 bpm or movement of chest wall with each breath. Prolonged inflation time (5-20 seconds) at 20-25 cm H_2O may overcome the long time constant of fluid-filled lungs for preterm infants
- Positive end-expiratory pressure (PEEP) during resuscitation improves oxygenation by maintaining functional residual capacity (FRC), improving respiratory compliance by 25% which reduces the need for intubation, mechanical ventilation, surfactant use and decreases the progression to respiratory distress syndrome (RDS). PPV can be easily provided with a flow-inflating bag or T-piece resuscitation device (but not with a self-inflating bag). With prolonged bag and mask ventilation, a nasal or orogastric tube should be inserted to decompress the stomach
- Administration of nasal continuous positive airway pressure (nCPAP) directly after resuscitation of infants breathing spontaneously with difficulty, is a gentle, efficient and noninvasive means to keep the lung open by maintaining lung volume, preventing lung atelectasis and stimulating respiration. This is associated with a reduction in the mortality of preterm infants but there may be an increased rate of pneumothorax. So spontaneously breathing preterm infants with respiratory distress may be supported with nCPAP or intubation and mechanical ventilation according to the administrator's expertise.

Assisted Ventilation Devices

The ability to provide consistent manual ventilation is dependent on the type of device:

- **Face mask with a self-inflating bag (Fig. 6.3)**: Self- inflating bags are without a manometer and a PEEP valve. They deliver required tidal volume but cannot deliver a constant PIP and an adequate PEEP. Pop – off valve is set to activate at a PIP of >40 cm of H_2O.

  Merits:
  - Ease of use
  - Easily available
  - Automatic re-expansion.

  Demerits:
  - False reassurance of ventilation as a large proportion of delivered breath may be unknowingly lost through leak around the mask.

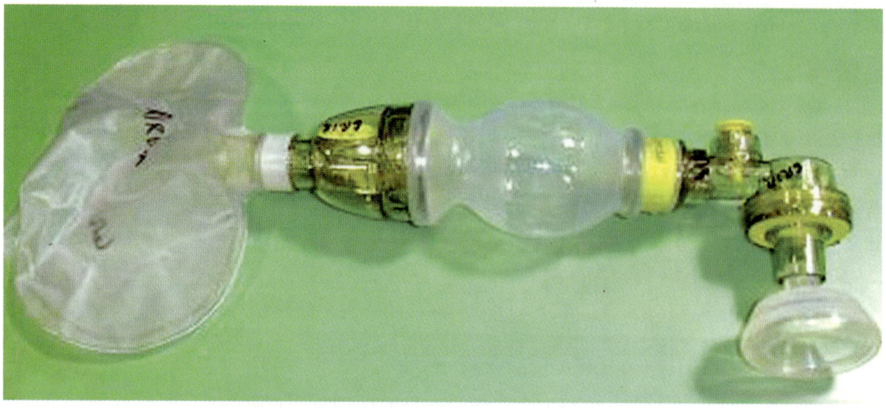

Fig. 6.3: Self-inflating bag with a reservoir

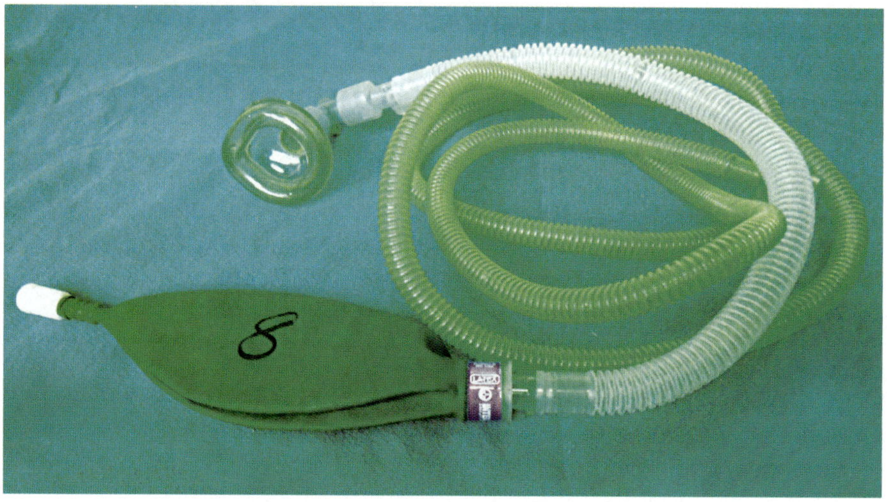

Fig. 6.4: Flow control bag

- These devices are unable to deliver consistent PIP, PEEP and prolonged inflation. They should not be used for ELBW infants.

• **Face mask with a flow-inflating bag (Fig. 6.4)**: They are technically challenging as the operator controls the volume and pressure of the bag by adjusting squeeze and egress at open end with fingers or flow control valve.

Merits:
- Possible to deliver oxygen concentration up to 100%.
- Higher PIP is possible as per requirement.

Demerits:
- Appropriate use requires adequate training and practice otherwise pressure may reach dangerously high level.
- Manometer needs to be continuously watched for safe PIP and consistent PEEP.
- Poor technique provides inconsistent PIP and PEEP.
- Maintaining constant PIP is difficult during a prolonged inflation of 5 seconds.

• **Face mask with a T-piece device (Fig. 6.5) (Neopuff™ Infant T-piece Resuscitator):** It is a pressure limited, mechanical T-piece resuscitation device with a variable PEEP valve, peak inspiratory pressure control and a manometer to show delivered pressure. The PIP and PEEP are preset and can be adjusted according to clinical response.

Merits:
- Easy to use even by relatively inexperienced operator.
- Best and easiest way to deliver a consistent and precise PIP, adequate PEEP and sustained inflation
- Produces significantly greater mean airway pressure.
- PIP and PEEP values provided are independent of user stress, fatigue level and skill.
- Operator has the advantage of observing the infant while providing ventilation as preset pressure is displayed on the manometer.
- Protects against the use of unintentional excess pressure.

Demerit:
- Expensive

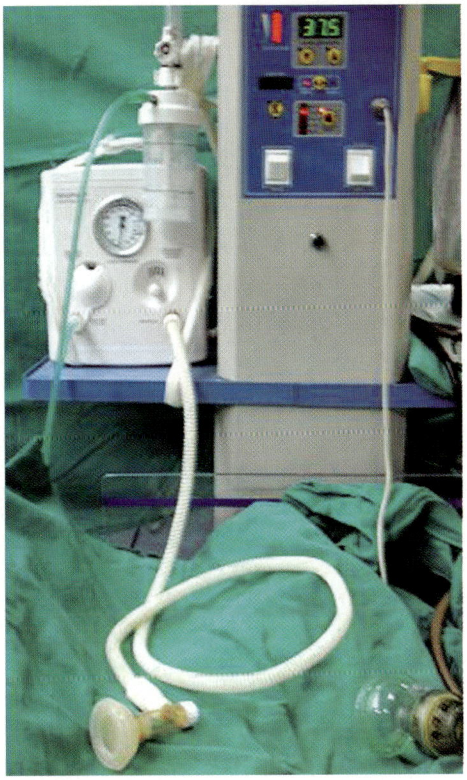

Fig. 6.5: Neopuff™ Infant T-piece Resuscitator

- Laryngeal mask airway (LMA) is indicated in resuscitation in situations such as failed bag and mask ventilation or failed intubation
- Endotracheal tube (ETT) intubation.

  Indications:
  - Initial endotracheal suctioning of non-vigorous meconium-stained babies
  - Ineffective bag and mask ventilation
  - Anticipated need for prolonged ventilation
  - When chest compressions are performed
  - As a route for emergency medication
  - Special resuscitative circumstances such as congenital diaphragmatic hernia, ELBW babies, etc.

A prompt increase in heart rate following intubation and PPV is the best indicator of correct placement of an ETT. Exhaled CO_2 detection is the recommended method of confirmation of ETT placement. It should be remembered that poor or absent pulmonary blood flow may give false-negative results which may lead to unnecessary extubation and reintubation of critically ill neonates with poor cardiac output.

CHEST COMPRESSIONS

Neonatal cardiac arrest is usually secondary to respiratory failure producing hypoxemia and tissue acidosis with resultant bradycardia, decreased cardiac contractility and eventually cardiac arrest. Thus, ventilation is the most effective step in neonatal resuscitation and chest compressions are likely to compete with effective ventilation, so the rescuers should always ensure optimal delivery of assisted ventilation before starting chest compressions. So the ABC resuscitation sequence is maintained except when the etiology is clearly cardiac.

- Compressions are indicated if heart rate is less than 60 bpm despite adequate ventilation with supplementary oxygen for 30 seconds.
- The two-finger technique or two thumb-encircling hands technique is used. The latter technique may generate higher peak systolic and coronary perfusion pressure and is recommended in newly borns. However, the two-finger technique is preferable when access to umbilicus is required during umbilical vessel catheterization. (Although it is possible to

use two-thumb-encircling hand technique in intubated infants with rescuer standing at baby's head thus permitting adequate access to umbilicus).
- The lower third of the sternum should be compressed to a depth of approximately one-third of the antero-posterior diameter of the chest.
- The recommended compression-to-ventilation ratio of 3:1 provides adequate minute ventilation which is critical for the vast majority of patients with asphyxial arrest. If the arrest is known to be of cardiac etiology, a higher ratio (15:2) for 2 rescuers should be considered.
- Coordinate with ventilation to avoid simultaneous delivery.
- The chest should be allowed to re-expand fully during relaxation, but the rescuer's thumbs should not leave the chest wall.
- Respiration, heart rate and oxygenation (optimally determined by pulse oximetry rather than assessment of color) should be reassessed periodically.
- Chest compressions should be stopped when heart rate is $\geq$60 bpm.
- Frequent interruptions of compressions should be avoided, as they will compromise artificial maintenance of systemic perfusion and coronary blood flow.

Medications: Drugs are rarely indicated because establishing adequate ventilation is the most important step towards correcting bradycardia in newly born.

Adrenaline: It is indicated if heart rate is less than 60 bpm despite adequate ventilation (usually with endotracheal intubation) with 100% oxygen and external cardiac compression for at least 30 seconds. If the heart rate still remains less than 60 bpm, it can be repeated every 3-5 minutes. The recommended route for administration is intravenous because of faster onset of action in comparison to the intratracheal route. The recommended intravenous concentration and dose is 1:10,000 (0.1 mg ml^{-1}) and 10-30 mcg kg^{-1} per dose respectively. Higher intravenous dose is not recommended because of exaggerated hypertension, decreased myocardial function and worse neurological function is seen in the dose range of 100 mcg kg^{-1}. While vascular access is being obtained, administration of a similar concentration, but higher dose (50-100 mcg kg^{-1}) through the ETT may be considered, but safety and effectiveness has not been evaluated.

VOLUME EXPANSION

Volume expansion is rarely indicated and restricted to situations where there is evidence of acute blood loss as in fetomaternal hemorrhage not responding adequately to other resuscitative measures and accompanied by clear signs of shock (pale skin, poor perfusion, weak pulse, persistent tachycardia, etc.). Isotonic crystalloid solution or blood is administered slowly as a 10 ml kg^{-1} bolus and can be repeated. In premature infants there is an increased risk of hypovolemia related to small blood volume. However, rapid volume expansion should be avoided in preterm babies because of their immature cerebral blood vessels which are more prone to intraventricular hemorrhage.

Post-resuscitation Care

Post-resuscitation care is necessary, as risk of deterioration exists even when their vital signs have returned to normal. Once adequate ventilation and circulation have been established, the infant should be nursed in an environment where close monitoring and anticipatory care can be provided.

1. *Glucose:* An association between hypoglycemia and a poor neurological outcome in perinatal asphyxia suggests to avoid low blood glucose level during resuscitation. Since no specific glucose level associated with worse outcome has been identified and hyperglycemia has been suggested as not harmful or rather protective by one recent pediatric series, intravenous glucose should be considered as soon as practical after resuscitation with the goal of avoiding hypoglycemia.
2. *Naloxone:* Naloxone hydrochloride is not recommended as part of initial resuscitative efforts in the delivery room for a newly born with respiratory depression. Heart rate and oxygenation should be restored by supporting ventilation. Naloxone can precipitate acute withdrawal and seizures in neonates of narcotic addicted mothers.
3. *Induced therapeutic hypothermia:* Infants born at ≥ 36 weeks gestation with evolving moderate to severe hypoxic ischemic encephalopathy should be offered therapeutic hypothermia as it significantly lowers morbidity (less neurodevelopmental disability) and mortality. The recommended protocol suggests hypothermia (33.5°C to 34.5°C) to commence within 6 hours following birth, to continue for 72 hours and to rewarm slowly over at least 4 hours. There may be some associated adverse effects such as thrombocytopenia and increased need for inotropic support.

GUIDELINES FOR WITHHOLDING OR DISCONTINUING RESUSCITATION

A consistent and coordinated approach to individual cases by the obstetric team, neonatology team and the parents is an important goal. Assessment of morbidity and mortality risks should be done with consideration of the available data and the changes in medical practice that may occur over time. Estimation of gestational age and birth weight should be accurate as even small discrepancies of 1 or 2 weeks between estimated and actual gestational age or a 100-200 gram difference in birth weight may have significant implications in terms of survival and long-term morbidity.

Withholding Resuscitation

Conditions associated with almost certain early mortality or unacceptably high morbidity in rare survivors, support non-initiation of resuscitation, e.g. anencephaly, gestational age < 23 weeks, birth weight <400 gm or chromosomal abnormalities such as trisomy 13, etc. However, in conditions associated with a high rate of survival and acceptable morbidity, resuscitation is nearly always indicated (i.e. gestational age ≥ 25 weeks, most congenital malformations). In conditions associated with uncertain prognosis, borderline survival, relatively high morbidity, anticipated high burden to the child, parental agreement concerning initiation of resuscitation should be supported.

Discontinuation of Resuscitation

Discontinuation of resuscitation may be justified if there is no sign of life (no heart beat and no respiratory effort) after 10 minutes of continuous and adequate resuscitative efforts as the subsequent end-point is either a high mortality or severe neurodevelopment disability. However, the decision to continue resuscitation beyond 10 minutes with no heart rate should consider the factors such as the presumed etiology of arrest, the gestational age, the potential role of therapeutic hypothermia and the parents' expressed feelings about the acceptable risk of morbidity.

Neonatal Resuscitation Equipment and Medications

1. *Suction equipment*
   - Meconium aspirator
   - Low pressure suction device
   - Bulb syringe
   - Suction catheters (5F,6F,8F)
   - 8F feeding tube and 20 ml syringe
2. *Bag and mask equipment*
   - Face mask sizes appropriate for newborn and premature babies
   - Oropharyngeal airway (30, 40, 50 mm)
   - Device to deliver 90-100% oxygen
   - Compressed air source
   - O_2 source with flow-meter (up to 10l/min)
   - Oxygen – air blender
   - Capnograph
   - LMA (size 1)
3. *Intubation equipment*
   - Straight – blade laryngoscope (preterm and term size)
   - Extra bulbs and batteries
   - Endotracheal tube (2-4 mm ID)
   - Stylet
   - Securing device for ETT
4. *Medications*
   - Epinephrine 1:10,000 (0.1 mg ml^{-1})
   - Isotonic normal saline/Ringer lactate

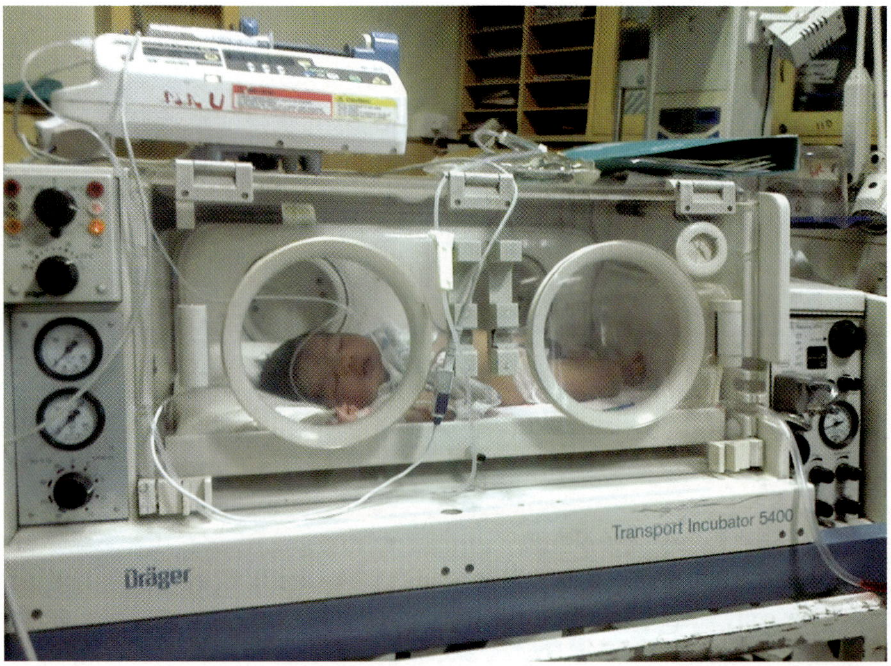

Fig. 6.6: Transport incubator

- Dextrose 10%
- Umbilical vessel catheterization tray and supplies

5. *Miscellaneous*
   - Gloves and personal protection items
   - Radiant warmer
   - Firm, padded resuscitation surface
   - Timer
   - Warmed linens
   - Stethoscope
   - Cardiac monitor
   - Pulse oximeter
6. *For very premature babies*
   - Plastic wrap
   - Transport incubator **(Fig. 6.6)**.

Index

Page numbers followed by *f* refer to figure and *t* refer to table, respectively.

T

U

V

W